Low-Sodium Diet Cookbook For Seniors

Complete Low-Sodium Foods For Seniors With Over 100 Recipes For Healthy Living

MONALISA BLAKE

0

TABLE OF CONTENT

INTRODUCTION

Sodium is a mineral that plays a crucial role in the human body's physiological functions. Found abundantly in nature and often consumed through various foods, sodium is essential for maintaining fluid balance, transmitting nerve impulses, and supporting muscle contractions. However, despite its importance, excessive sodium intake can have detrimental effects on health, particularly concerning cardiovascular health and blood pressure regulation, bto comprehend the significance of sodium in the body, it's essential to delve into its physiological functions. Sodium primarily exists in the extracellular fluid, where it helps regulate osmotic pressure and maintain proper hydration levels. Alongside other electrolytes like potassium and chloride, sodium facilitates the transmission of nerve signals and muscle contractions, ensuring vital bodily processes function smoothly. Without adequate sodium intake, individuals may experience symptoms such as muscle weakness, fatigue, and impaired cognitive function.

Despite its critical role, excessive sodium consumption has emerged as a significant public health concern, particularly due to its association with hypertension, or high blood pressure. Hypertension affects millions of individuals worldwide and is a leading risk factor for cardiovascular diseases such as heart attacks and strokes. The link between sodium intake and blood pressure levels has been extensively studied, with research consistently indicating that high sodium diets can elevate blood pressure, thereby increasing the risk of cardiovascular complications.

The mechanisms underlying sodium's impact on blood pressure are multifaceted. One key factor is sodium's ability to increase extracellular fluid volume, leading to higher blood volume and subsequently raising blood pressure. Additionally, sodium promotes the constriction of blood vessels, further contributing to elevated blood pressure levels. Over time, chronic hypertension can damage blood vessels and organs, including the heart, brain, and kidneys, posing significant health risks, especially for older adults.

Seniors, in particular, are susceptible to the adverse effects of high sodium intake due to age-related changes in the body's ability to regulate sodium balance. As individuals age, kidney function may decline, impairing the body's ability to excrete excess sodium efficiently. Moreover, aging is often accompanied by changes in taste perception and dietary habits, potentially leading to increased sodium consumption. Consequently, seniors must be vigilant about monitoring their sodium intake and adopting strategies to reduce its adverse effects on their health.

A critical aspect of sodium management involves understanding the sources of dietary sodium. While table salt is a well-known contributor, many processed and packaged foods contain high levels of sodium as well. These hidden sources of sodium, including canned soups, processed meats, and fast food, can significantly contribute to daily sodium intake without individuals realizing it. Therefore, reading food labels and making informed choices at the grocery store are essential steps in reducing sodium consumption.

The benefits of adopting a low-sodium diet extend beyond blood pressure management to encompass overall cardiovascular health and well-being. Research suggests that reducing sodium intake can lead to improvements in blood pressure control, reducing the risk of heart disease and stroke. Additionally, a low-sodium diet may have positive effects on other health parameters, such as kidney function and bone health, further emphasizing its importance for seniors' overall health.

Implementing a low-sodium diet requires practical strategies and lifestyle modifications. These may include cooking at home using fresh ingredients, incorporating herbs and spices for flavor, and limiting the consumption of processed and restaurant foods. Furthermore, individuals can benefit from monitoring their sodium intake through food journals or smartphone apps, enabling them to track their progress and make adjustments as needed.

Importance of a Low-Sodium Diet for Seniors

Sodium, a mineral commonly found in many foods, can have significant implications for seniors' health, especially concerning cardiovascular health, blood pressure management, and overall well-being. One of the primary reasons why a low-sodium diet is essential for seniors is its impact on blood pressure regulation. Hypertension, or high blood pressure, is a prevalent health condition among older adults and is a leading risk factor for cardiovascular diseases such as heart attacks and strokes. Excessive sodium consumption can contribute to elevated blood pressure levels, increasing the risk of hypertension and its associated complications. By reducing sodium intake, seniors can help maintain healthy blood pressure levels and mitigate the risk of cardiovascular diseases.

Furthermore, seniors may be more susceptible to the adverse effects of high sodium intake due to age-related changes in the body's ability to regulate sodium balance. As individuals age, kidney function may decline, impairing the body's ability to excrete excess sodium efficiently. Additionally, seniors may experience alterations in taste perception and dietary habits, potentially leading to increased sodium consumption. Therefore, adopting a low-sodium diet is essential for supporting optimal kidney function and minimizing the risk of sodium-related health complications in older adults.

In addition to its impact on blood pressure and kidney function, reducing sodium intake can have broader implications for seniors' overall health and well-being. Excessive sodium consumption has been linked to other health conditions beyond hypertension, including osteoporosis, stomach cancer, and cognitive decline. By adopting a low-sodium diet, seniors can help reduce their risk of developing these conditions and promote better long-term health outcomes.

Seniors may benefit from a low-sodium diet in managing other chronic health conditions commonly associated with aging, such as diabetes and heart disease. High sodium intake can exacerbate existing health issues and complicate disease management efforts. By reducing sodium intake and focusing on whole, nutrient-dense foods, seniors can better control their health conditions and improve their quality of life.

Implementing a low-sodium diet does not mean sacrificing flavor or enjoyment in meals. Seniors can still enjoy delicious and satisfying foods while prioritizing their health through mindful food choices and cooking techniques. Incorporating flavorful herbs, spices, and other seasonings can enhance the taste of meals without relying on excessive salt. Additionally, choosing fresh, whole foods over processed and packaged options can significantly reduce sodium intake while providing essential nutrients and promoting overall health.

How This Cookbook Can Help

This cookbook serves as a valuable resource for seniors looking to improve their health and well-being through dietary changes, specifically by adopting a low-sodium diet. By providing a wide range of delicious and nutritious recipes, along with practical tips and guidance, this cookbook aims to empower seniors to make informed choices about their dietary habits and take proactive steps towards better health outcomes.

One of the primary ways in which this cookbook can help seniors is by offering a diverse selection of low-sodium recipes that are both flavorful and satisfying. Many seniors may be accustomed to traditional cooking methods that rely heavily on salt for seasoning. However, by introducing alternative herbs, spices, and seasonings, this cookbook demonstrates how to enhance the taste of meals without the need for excessive salt. From breakfast delights to decadent desserts, each recipe is carefully crafted to prioritize flavor while adhering to low-sodium guidelines, ensuring that seniors can enjoy delicious meals without compromising their health.

In addition to providing delicious recipes, this cookbook also offers practical guidance on how to navigate the grocery store and choose low-sodium ingredients. Many processed and packaged foods contain high levels of hidden sodium, making it challenging for seniors to identify suitable options for their dietary needs. By educating readers about common sources of dietary sodium and offering tips for reading food labels, this cookbook equips seniors with the knowledge and skills they need to make healthier choices while shopping for groceries. Furthermore, by highlighting the importance of fresh, whole foods in a low-sodium diet, this cookbook encourages seniors to prioritize nutrient-dense ingredients and minimize their reliance on processed foods.

This cookbook serves as a comprehensive guide to meal planning and preparation, offering practical strategies for incorporating low-sodium meals into seniors' daily routines. From batch cooking techniques to weekly meal plans, seniors will find helpful tips and suggestions for simplifying meal preparation and saving time in the kitchen. By emphasizing the importance of planning ahead and preparing meals in advance, this cookbook empowers seniors to maintain a consistent low-sodium diet without feeling overwhelmed or burdened by the demands of daily cooking.

Moreover, this cookbook recognizes that adopting a low-sodium diet is not just about following recipes but also about making sustainable lifestyle changes that promote long-term health and well-being. Therefore, in addition to offering delicious recipes and practical tips, this cookbook also provides guidance on overcoming common challenges and staying motivated on the low-sodium journey. Whether it's dealing with social situations that involve food or coping with cravings and temptations, seniors will find helpful strategies and encouragement to help them stay on track and achieve their health goals.

CHAPTER ONE:

Sodium in common foods

Understanding the sodium content in common foods is essential for seniors aiming to reduce their sodium intake. Here's a breakdown of the sodium levels in various food categories, categorized as low, medium, and high:

Low Sodium Foods (0-140 mg per serving):

- Fresh fruits and vegetables (e.g., apples, oranges, broccoli, spinach)
- Whole grains and legumes (e.g., brown rice, quinoa, lentils)
- Lean proteins (e.g., skinless chicken breast, tofu, fish)
- Herbs and spices (e.g., basil, oregano, garlic powder)
- Unsweetened dairy products (e.g., plain yogurt, milk, cheese)
- Nuts and seeds (e.g., almonds, chia seeds, sunflower seeds)
- Condiments and seasonings (e.g., vinegar, mustard, lemon juice)

Medium Sodium Foods (140-400 mg per serving):

- Whole grain bread and cereals (e.g., whole wheat bread, oatmeal)
- Canned vegetables (e.g., canned tomatoes, green beans)
- Processed meats (e.g., turkey deli meat, canned tuna)
- Cheese (e.g., cheddar cheese, feta cheese)
- Soups and broths (e.g., low-sodium canned soups, homemade broth)
- Plant-based meat alternatives (e.g., tofu hot dogs, veggie burgers)
- Breakfast cereals (e.g., bran flakes, corn flakes)

High Sodium Foods (400+ mg per serving):

- Processed and cured meats (e.g., bacon, ham, sausage)
- Canned soups and sauces (e.g., canned chili, spaghetti sauce)
- Frozen meals and convenience foods (e.g., frozen pizza, TV dinners)
- Snack foods (e.g., potato chips, pretzels, salted nuts)
- Processed cheese products (e.g., cheese slices, cheese spreads)
- Pickled and fermented foods (e.g., pickles, olives, sauerkraut)

- Condiments and sauces (e.g., soy sauce, ketchup, barbecue sauce)

When selecting foods for a low-sodium diet, seniors should prioritize options from the low sodium category and limit their consumption of medium and high sodium foods. Additionally, seniors should be mindful of portion sizes and avoid adding extra salt during cooking or at the table. By incorporating more low sodium options into their diet and reducing their intake of high sodium foods, seniors can effectively manage their sodium consumption and improve their overall health and well-being.

Assessing Current Sodium Intake

Assessing current sodium intake is an essential first step for seniors who are considering transitioning to a low-sodium diet. By understanding their baseline sodium consumption, seniors can identify areas for improvement and set realistic goals for sodium reduction. Here are some practical methods for assessing current sodium intake:

1. Food Journaling: Keeping a detailed food journal is one of the most effective ways to assess current sodium intake. Seniors can record everything they eat and drink over several days, including meals, snacks, and beverages. It's essential to note portion sizes and preparation methods, as these factors can significantly impact sodium content. By reviewing the food journal, seniors can gain insight into their typical dietary patterns and identify sources of high sodium consumption.

2. Reviewing Food Labels: Seniors can evaluate the sodium content of foods by reviewing nutrition labels on packaged products. Paying attention to the sodium content per serving size is crucial, as many packaged foods contain multiple **Servings** per container. It's essential to be mindful of hidden sources of sodium, such as added salt, sodium-based preservatives, and flavor enhancers. By reviewing food labels, seniors can identify high sodium items in their diet and make informed choices when selecting groceries.

3. Sodium Tracking Apps: Utilizing smartphone apps designed for tracking nutrition can streamline the process of assessing sodium intake. These apps typically have extensive databases of food items and their corresponding sodium content, allowing seniors to log their meals and monitor their sodium consumption more efficiently. Some apps also provide insights into overall dietary patterns and nutrient intake, helping seniors make informed decisions about their eating habits.

4. Dietary Recall Interviews: Seniors can participate in dietary recall interviews conducted by healthcare professionals or registered dietitians. During these interviews, seniors are asked to recall everything they ate and drank over a specified period, typically the previous 24 hours. Healthcare professionals can then analyze the dietary recall data to assess sodium intake and provide personalized recommendations for sodium reduction.

5. Sodium Excretion Tests: In some cases, healthcare providers may recommend sodium excretion tests to assess sodium intake more accurately. These tests measure the amount of sodium excreted in urine over a specified period, providing insights into overall sodium consumption. While sodium excretion tests offer a more objective assessment of sodium intake, they are typically reserved for research purposes or individuals with specific medical conditions.

Setting Personalized Sodium Goals

Setting personalized sodium goals is a crucial step for seniors embarking on a low-sodium diet journey. By establishing realistic and achievable targets based on individual health needs, seniors can effectively manage their sodium intake and work towards improving their overall well-being. Here are some steps to help seniors set personalized sodium goals:

1. Consultation with Healthcare Professionals: Seniors should consult with their healthcare provider or a registered dietitian to determine appropriate sodium goals based on their specific health status and medical history. Healthcare professionals can assess individual risk factors, such as hypertension, kidney disease, and heart conditions, and provide personalized recommendations for sodium intake.

2. Understanding Sodium Recommendations: Seniors should familiarize themselves with current dietary guidelines and recommendations for sodium intake. According to the Dietary Guidelines for Americans, the general recommendation for adults is to consume less than 2,300 milligrams of sodium per day, with an ideal limit of 1,500 milligrams per day for certain population groups, including adults over the age of 51, individuals with hypertension, diabetes, or chronic kidney disease. Seniors should consider these guidelines when setting their personalized sodium goals.

3. Assessing Baseline Sodium Intake: Seniors should assess their current sodium intake using methods such as food journaling, reviewing food labels, or utilizing smartphone apps designed for tracking nutrition. By understanding their baseline sodium consumption, seniors can identify areas for improvement and set realistic goals for sodium reduction.

4. Gradual Reduction Approach: Seniors may find it beneficial to adopt a gradual reduction approach when setting sodium goals. Rather than attempting to drastically reduce sodium intake overnight, seniors can set incremental goals and make gradual changes to their dietary habits over time. For example, seniors may start by gradually reducing the amount of salt added during cooking and at the table, substituting high-sodium condiments with lower sodium alternatives, and gradually transitioning to low-sodium versions of their favorite foods.

5. Personal Preferences and Dietary Patterns: Seniors should consider their personal preferences and dietary patterns when setting sodium goals. It's essential to choose strategies that are sustainable and align with individual tastes and lifestyle preferences. Seniors may find it helpful to experiment with different cooking techniques, seasonings, and flavor enhancers to make low-sodium meals more enjoyable and satisfying.

6. Monitoring and Adjustments: Seniors should regularly monitor their sodium intake and make adjustments to their goals as needed. By tracking their progress over time, seniors can identify patterns and trends in their dietary habits and make informed decisions about their sodium consumption. Seniors should be flexible and willing to make adjustments based on their individual needs and preferences.

7. Celebrating Progress: Seniors should celebrate milestones achieved on their low-sodium journey and reward themselves for sticking to their goals. Celebrating progress, no matter how small, can help seniors stay motivated and committed to their dietary goals. Seniors should acknowledge their achievements and use them as motivation to continue making positive changes to their diet and lifestyle.

Tips for Reading Food Labels

1. Pay Attention to Serving Size: The serving size listed on the nutrition label is critical as all the nutrient information provided is based on this serving size. Seniors should compare the serving size listed on the label to the portion they typically consume to ensure accuracy.

2. Check the Sodium Content: Look for the sodium content per serving size. Seniors should aim for foods with lower sodium levels. Foods with 5% Daily Value (DV) or less of sodium per serving are considered low in sodium, while those with 20% DV or more are high in sodium.

3. Look for Hidden Sodium Sources: Sodium can hide in various forms, including sodium-based preservatives (e.g., monosodium glutamate or MSG), sodium bicarbonate (baking soda), and sodium nitrate/nitrite. Seniors should scan the ingredient list for these additives and be cautious of products containing them.

4. Beware of "Sodium-Free" vs. "No Added Salt": "Sodium-free" on a label means the product contains less than 5 milligrams of sodium per serving. "No added salt" indicates that the product was made without additional salt during processing, but it may still contain natural sodium. Seniors should distinguish between these terms when selecting low-sodium options.

5. Choose Whole Foods: Whole, unprocessed foods typically contain lower levels of sodium compared to processed and packaged foods. Seniors should prioritize fresh fruits and vegetables, lean proteins, whole grains, and unsalted nuts and seeds.

6. Be Wary of Common High-Sodium Culprits: Certain foods tend to be higher in sodium, such as canned soups, processed meats, salty snacks, and condiments like soy sauce and ketchup. Seniors should limit their consumption of these high-sodium items and opt for lower sodium alternatives when available.

7. Compare Products: Seniors can compare similar products to choose the option with the lower sodium content. Some products offer reduced-sodium or sodium-free versions, which can be healthier alternatives.

8. Consider the %DV: The % Daily Value (%DV) listed on the nutrition label indicates how much of the recommended daily intake of a nutrient one serving provides. Seniors can use the %DV to assess whether a food is high or low in sodium compared to their daily sodium goals.

9. Use Online Resources and Apps: There are online databases and smartphone apps that provide extensive information about the sodium content of various foods. Seniors can use these resources to research and plan low-sodium meals and verify the sodium content of foods not found in traditional databases.

10. Be Mindful of Health Claims: While terms like "low-sodium," "reduced sodium," and "no added salt" may appear on food packaging, seniors should still check the actual sodium content on the nutrition label. Some products may still contain significant amounts of sodium despite these claims.

CHAPTER TWO:

Essential Ingredients for a Low-Sodium Kitchen

1. **Herbs and Spices:** Herbs and spices are excellent alternatives to salt for enhancing the flavor of dishes. Stock up on a variety of options such as:

   - Basil

   - Oregano

   - Thyme

   - Rosemary

   - Cumin

   - Paprika

   - Turmeric

   - Garlic powder

   - Onion powder

2. **Citrus Fruits:** Citrus fruits like lemons, limes, and oranges can add brightness and acidity to dishes without the need for salt. Use them to season salads, marinades, and dressings.

3. **Vinegars:** Vinegars, such as balsamic vinegar, apple cider vinegar, and rice vinegar, can add tanginess to dishes and enhance their flavor profile. They're great for making low-sodium vinaigrettes and sauces.

4. **Low-Sodium Broths and Stocks:** Opt for low-sodium or sodium-free versions of broths and stocks to use as a base for soups, stews, and sauces. Look for options labeled "reduced sodium" or "no salt added."

5. **Sodium-Free Seasoning Blends:** Some companies offer seasoning blends specifically formulated to be sodium-free. These blends often contain a mix of herbs, spices, and other flavorings to add depth to dishes.

6. **Unsalted Nuts and Seeds:** Nuts and seeds are nutritious snacks and ingredients for cooking and baking. Look for unsalted varieties such as almonds, walnuts, pumpkin seeds, and sunflower seeds.

7. **Whole Grains:** Whole grains like brown rice, quinoa, barley, and oats are naturally low in sodium and high in fiber. They're versatile ingredients that can be used in various dishes, from salads to casseroles.

8. **Legumes:** Beans, lentils, and chickpeas are excellent sources of protein, fiber, and nutrients. They're low in sodium when cooked from dried or canned without added salt. Use them in soups, salads, and main dishes.

9. **Fresh Produce:** Fresh fruits and vegetables are naturally low in sodium and rich in vitamins, minerals, and antioxidants. Incorporate a variety of colorful produce into your meals to add flavor, texture, and nutrition.

10. **Low-Sodium Condiments:** Look for low-sodium versions of condiments such as mustard, ketchup, soy sauce, and salsa. These alternatives provide flavor without the excessive sodium content found in regular condiments.

11. **Healthy Fats:** Incorporate healthy fats like olive oil, avocado oil, and coconut oil into your cooking and meal preparation. These fats add richness and flavor to dishes without contributing to sodium levels.

12. **Plain Yogurt and Cottage Cheese:** Choose plain, unsweetened yogurt and cottage cheese as alternatives to high-sodium dairy products. They can be used in both savory and sweet recipes, from dips to desserts.

Herbs, Spices, and Seasonings

Herbs:

1. Basil
2. Parsley
3. Cilantro
4. Dill
5. Mint
6. Chives
7. Sage
8. Rosemary
9. Thyme
10. Oregano
11. Tarragon
12. Bay leaves
13. Marjoram

14. Lemongrass

15. Lavender

16. Fennel fronds

Spices:

1. Cumin

2. Paprika (smoked or sweet)

3. Chili powder

4. Turmeric

5. Coriander

6. Ginger (ground or fresh)

7. Cinnamon

8. Nutmeg

9. Cloves

10. Allspice

11. Cardamom

12. Mustard powder

13. Cayenne pepper

14. Black pepper (freshly ground)

15. White pepper

16. Saffron

Seasoning Blends:

1. Italian seasoning

2. Herbes de Provence

3. Curry powder

4. Garam masala

5. Taco seasoning (homemade, low-sodium)

6. Cajun seasoning (homemade, low-sodium)

7. Chinese five-spice

8. Ras el hanout

9. Za'atar

10. Everything bagel seasoning (homemade, low-sodium)

11. Lemon pepper seasoning (homemade, low-sodium)

12. Ranch seasoning (homemade, low-sodium)

13. Poultry seasoning

14. Steak seasoning (homemade, low-sodium)

15. Adobo seasoning (homemade, low-sodium)

Low-Sodium Cooking Oils

When selecting cooking oils for a low-sodium diet, it's essential to choose options that are naturally low in sodium and contain healthy fats. Here are some low-sodium cooking oils to consider:

1. **Olive Oil:** Extra virgin olive oil is a popular choice for cooking and dressing salads. It's rich in monounsaturated fats and antioxidants, making it a heart-healthy option. Look for cold-pressed or unrefined varieties for the most flavor and nutritional benefits.

2. **Avocado Oil:** Avocado oil has a high smoke point, making it suitable for high-heat cooking methods like sautéing, frying, and grilling. It's rich in monounsaturated fats and contains beneficial nutrients like vitamin E and antioxidants.

3. **Coconut Oil:** Virgin coconut oil is a flavorful option for cooking and baking. While it's higher in saturated fat compared to other oils, it can still be part of a balanced diet when used in moderation. Look for unrefined or cold-pressed coconut oil for the most flavor and nutritional benefits.

4. **Canola Oil:** Canola oil is a versatile and neutral-flavored oil that's suitable for various cooking methods, including sautéing, baking, and frying. It's low in saturated fat and contains heart-healthy omega-3 fatty acids.

5. **Grapeseed Oil:** Grapeseed oil has a high smoke point, making it ideal for high-heat cooking methods like stir-frying and deep-frying. It's also relatively neutral in flavor, making it suitable for a wide range of dishes.

6. **Sunflower Oil:** Sunflower oil is another option with a high smoke point, making it suitable for frying and other high-heat cooking methods. It's rich in vitamin E and contains heart-healthy monounsaturated and polyunsaturated fats.

7. **Sesame Oil:** Sesame oil adds a unique flavor to dishes and is commonly used in Asian cuisine. It's best used in small amounts as a finishing oil or for light sautéing due to its strong flavor. Look for toasted sesame oil for a more intense flavor profile.

8. **Walnut Oil:** Walnut oil has a rich, nutty flavor and is best used as a finishing oil for salads, dressings, and drizzling over cooked dishes. It's high in omega-3 fatty acids and contains beneficial antioxidants.

Sodium-Free Broths and Stocks

1. **Homemade Broth or Stock:** Making your own broth or stock allows you to control the sodium content entirely. Simply simmer vegetables (such as onions, carrots, celery, and herbs) in water for a vegetable broth or add bones or meat for a meat-based stock. You can customize the flavor with herbs, spices, and aromatics to suit your taste preferences.

2. **Sodium-Free Broth Bases:** Some specialty stores or online retailers offer sodium-free broth bases or bouillon cubes. These products are typically made without added salt and can be dissolved in water to create a flavorful broth or stock. Look for options labeled as "sodium-free" or "no salt added."

3. **Vegetable Juices:** Vegetable juices like tomato juice or carrot juice can serve as a base for sodium-free broths or stocks. Simply dilute the vegetable juice with water to achieve the desired consistency and flavor. You can also enhance the flavor with herbs, spices, and other seasonings.

4. **Homemade Vegetable Purees:** Pureeing cooked vegetables with water can create a flavorful base for sodium-free broths or stocks. Simply blend cooked vegetables (such as tomatoes, carrots, onions, and garlic) with water until smooth, then strain the mixture to remove any solids. Adjust the seasoning with herbs, spices, and other flavorings as desired.

5. **Water:** In some recipes, especially those with other flavorful ingredients, plain water can serve as a suitable substitute for broth or stock. While it may not add the same depth of flavor, water can still provide moisture and help bind ingredients together in dishes like soups, stews, and sauces.

CHAPTER THREE:

Breakfast Delights

Apple-Chai Smoothie:

Prep Time: 5 minutes

Servings: 2

Ingredients:

- 2 large apples, cored and chopped
- 1 cup unsweetened almond milk
- 1/2 cup plain Greek yogurt
- 1 teaspoon chai spice blend (or a combination of cinnamon, cardamom, ginger, cloves, and nutmeg)
- 1 tablespoon honey or maple syrup (optional, for sweetness)
- Ice cubes (optional)

Instructions:

1. In a blender, combine the chopped apples, almond milk, Greek yogurt, chai spice blend, and honey or maple syrup (if using).
2. Blend until smooth and creamy, adding ice cubes if desired for a colder consistency.
3. Pour the smoothie into glasses.
4. Serve immediately and enjoy!

Nutritional Values (Approximate, per serving):

- Calories: 80-100 kcal
- Protein: 2-3 grams
- Fat: 4-6 grams
- Saturated Fat: 1 gram
- Carbohydrates: 10-12 grams
- Dietary Fiber: 2-3 grams
- Sugars: 6-8 grams

Blueberry-Pineapple Smoothie:

Prep Time: 5 minutes

Servings: 2

Ingredients:

- 1 cup blueberries (fresh or frozen)
- 1 cup pineapple chunks (fresh or frozen)
- 1 banana, peeled and sliced
- 1/2 cup plain Greek yogurt
- 1/2 cup unsweetened almond milk
- 1 tablespoon honey or maple syrup (optional, for sweetness)
- Ice cubes (optional)
- Fresh blueberries and pineapple wedges, for garnish

Instructions:

1. In a blender, combine the blueberries, pineapple chunks, banana slices, Greek yogurt, almond milk, and honey or maple syrup (if using).
2. Blend until smooth and creamy, adding ice cubes if desired for a colder consistency.
3. Pour the smoothie into glasses.
4. Garnish with fresh blueberries and pineapple wedges.
5. Serve immediately and enjoy!

Nutritional Values (Approximate, per serving):

- Calories: 150-200 kcal
- Protein: 8-10 grams
- Fat: 2-3 grams
- Saturated Fat: 0 grams
- Carbohydrates: 30-35 grams
- Dietary Fiber: 4-6 grams
- Sugars: 20-25 grams

Watermelon-Raspberry Smoothie:

Prep Time: 5 minutes

Servings: 2

Ingredients:

- 2 cups cubed watermelon
- 1 cup raspberries (fresh or frozen)
- 1/2 cup plain Greek yogurt
- 1/2 cup coconut water or water
- 1 tablespoon honey or maple syrup (optional, for sweetness)
- Ice cubes (optional)
- Fresh mint leaves and watermelon slices, for garnish

Instructions:

1. In a blender, combine the watermelon cubes, raspberries, Greek yogurt, coconut water or water, and honey or maple syrup (if using).
2. Blend until smooth and creamy, adding ice cubes if desired for a colder consistency.
3. Pour the smoothie into glasses.
4. Garnish with fresh mint leaves and watermelon slices.
5. Serve immediately and enjoy!

Nutritional Values (Approximate, per serving):

- Calories: 100-150 kcal
- Protein: 4-6 grams
- Fat: 1-2 grams
- Saturated Fat: 0 grams
- Carbohydrates: 20-25 grams
- Dietary Fiber: 3-5 grams
- Sugars: 15-20 grams

Festive Berry Parfait:

Prep Time: 10 minutes

Servings: 2

Ingredients:

- 1 cup mixed berries (such as strawberries, blueberries, raspberries)
- 1 cup plain Greek yogurt
- 1/2 cup granola
- 2 tablespoons honey or maple syrup (optional, for sweetness)
- Fresh mint leaves and additional berries, for garnish

Instructions:

1. In two serving glasses or bowls, layer the mixed berries, Greek yogurt, and granola.
2. Drizzle honey or maple syrup over each parfait layer if desired.
3. Repeat the layers until glasses are filled, ending with a layer of berries and a sprinkle of granola on top.
4. Garnish with fresh mint leaves and additional berries.
5. Serve immediately as a festive and nutritious breakfast or dessert option.

Nutritional Values (Approximate, per serving):

- Calories: 250-300 kcal
- Protein: 15-20 grams
- Fat: 5-7 grams
- Saturated Fat: 1-2 grams
- Carbohydrates: 30-35 grams
- Dietary Fiber: 5-7 grams
- Sugars: 15-20 grams

Mixed-Grain Hot Cereal:

Prep Time: 10 minutes   **Cook Time:** 20 minutes   **Servings:** 4

Ingredients:

- 1/2 cup rolled oats
- 1/4 cup quinoa
- 1/4 cup barley
- 1/4 cup millet
- 2 cups water
- 2 cups milk (dairy or plant-based)
- 1/4 teaspoon salt
- Optional toppings: sliced bananas, berries, nuts, honey or maple syrup

Instructions:

1. In a medium saucepan, combine the rolled oats, quinoa, barley, millet, water, milk, and salt.

2. Bring the mixture to a boil over medium heat, then reduce the heat to low and simmer for about 15-20 minutes, stirring occasionally, until the grains are tender and the mixture has thickened.

3. Once cooked, remove the hot cereal from the heat and let it sit for a few minutes to thicken further.

4. Serve the hot cereal in bowls, topped with sliced bananas, berries, nuts, and a drizzle of honey or maple syrup if desired.

5. Enjoy this wholesome and nutritious mixed-grain hot cereal for a hearty breakfast!

Nutritional Values (Approximate, per serving):

- Calories: 200-250 kcal
- Protein: 8-10 grams
- Fat: 4-6 grams
- Saturated Fat: 1-2 grams
- Carbohydrates: 30-35 grams

- Dietary Fiber: 4-6 grams

- Sugars: 4-6 grams

Corn Pudding:

Prep Time: 10 minutes
Cook Time: 45 minutes
Servings: 6

Ingredients:

- 2 cups corn kernels (fresh or frozen)

- 1 cup milk (dairy or plant-based)

- 3 eggs

- 1/4 cup melted butter or margarine

- 1/4 cup all-purpose flour

- 1/4 cup sugar

- 1/2 teaspoon salt

Instructions:

1. Preheat your oven to 350°F (175°C). Grease a baking dish.

2. In a blender, combine the corn kernels, milk, eggs, melted butter, flour, sugar, and salt. Blend until smooth.

3. Pour the mixture into the prepared baking dish.

4. Bake for 40-45 minutes, or until the pudding is set and lightly golden on top.

5. Allow the pudding to cool slightly before serving.

6. Serve warm as a comforting side dish or dessert.

Nutritional Values (Approximate, per serving):

- Calories: 200-250 kcal

- Protein: 6-8 grams

- Fat: 8-10 grams

- Saturated Fat: 4-6 grams

- Carbohydrates: 25-30 grams

- Dietary Fiber: 2-3 grams

- Sugars: 8-10 grams

Rhubarb Bread Pudding:

Prep Time: 15 minutes
Cook Time: 45 minutes
Servings: 8

Ingredients:

- 4 cups cubed bread (day-old or slightly stale)

- 2 cups chopped rhubarb

- 4 eggs

- 2 cups milk (dairy or plant-based)

- 1/2 cup sugar

- 1 teaspoon vanilla extract

- 1/2 teaspoon ground cinnamon

- Pinch of salt

Instructions:

1. Preheat your oven to 350°F (175°C). Grease a baking dish.

2. In a large bowl, combine the cubed bread and chopped rhubarb.

3. In another bowl, whisk together the eggs, milk, sugar, vanilla extract, cinnamon, and salt.

4. Pour the egg mixture over the bread and rhubarb, stirring gently to coat.

5. Let the mixture sit for about 10-15 minutes to allow the bread to absorb the liquid.

6. Pour the bread pudding mixture into the prepared baking dish.

7. Bake for 40-45 minutes, or until the pudding is set and golden on top.

8. Allow the pudding to cool slightly before serving.

9. Serve warm as a delightful dessert or brunch dish.

Nutritional Values (Approximate, per serving):

- Calories: 250-300 kcal

- Protein: 8-10 grams

- Fat: 8-10 grams

- Saturated Fat: 3-5 grams

- Carbohydrates: 35-40 grams

- Dietary Fiber: 2-3 grams

- Sugars: 15-20 grams

Cinnamon-Nutmeg Blueberry Muffins:

Prep	**Time:**	15	minutes
Cook	**Time:**	20	minutes

Servings: 12

Ingredients:

- 2 cups all-purpose flour

- 1/2 cup sugar

- 2 teaspoons baking powder

- 1/2 teaspoon baking soda

- 1/2 teaspoon salt

- 1 teaspoon ground cinnamon

- 1/2 teaspoon ground nutmeg

- 1 cup blueberries (fresh or frozen)

- 2 large eggs

- 1 cup buttermilk

- 1/2 cup unsalted butter, melted

- 1 teaspoon vanilla extract

Instructions:

1. Preheat your oven to 375°F (190°C). Line a muffin tin with paper liners.

2. In a large bowl, whisk together the flour, sugar, baking powder, baking soda, salt, cinnamon, and nutmeg.

3. Gently fold in the blueberries until evenly distributed.

4. In another bowl, whisk together the eggs, buttermilk, melted butter, and vanilla extract.

5. Pour the wet ingredients into the dry ingredients and stir until just combined. Do not overmix; it's okay if the batter is slightly lumpy.

6. Divide the batter evenly among the muffin cups, filling each about two-thirds full.

7. Bake for 18-20 minutes, or until the muffins are golden brown and a toothpick inserted into the center comes out clean.

8. Remove the muffins from the oven and let them cool in the tin for a few minutes before transferring to a wire rack to cool completely.

9. Serve the muffins warm or at room temperature, and enjoy!

Nutritional Values (Approximate, per serving):

- Calories: 180-200 kcal

- Protein: 4-6 grams

- Fat: 8-10 grams

- Saturated Fat: 5-7 grams

- Carbohydrates: 25-30 grams

- Dietary Fiber: 1-2 grams

- Sugars: 10-12 grams

Prep **Time:** 5 minutes
Cook **Time:** 5 minutes
Servings: 1

Ingredients:

- 1 whole wheat or multigrain tortilla
- 1/4 cup sliced strawberries
- 1/4 cup blueberries
- 1/4 cup diced apple
- 1/4 cup shredded cheddar cheese
- 1 tablespoon honey or maple syrup (optional)

Instructions:

1. Place the tortilla on a flat surface.
2. Sprinkle the shredded cheddar cheese evenly over the tortilla.
3. Arrange the sliced strawberries, blueberries, and diced apple over one half of the tortilla.
4. Drizzle honey or maple syrup over the fruit if desired.
5. Fold the empty half of the tortilla over the fruit and cheese to form a wrap.
6. Heat a skillet over medium heat and place the breakfast wrap seam-side down.
7. Cook for 2-3 minutes on each side, or until the tortilla is golden brown and the cheese is melted.
8. Remove from the skillet and let cool for a minute before slicing.
9. Serve warm and enjoy this fruity and cheesy breakfast wrap!

Nutritional Values (Approximate, per serving):

- Calories: 250-300 kcal
- Protein: 8-10 grams
- Fat: 8-10 grams
- Saturated Fat: 4-6 grams
- Carbohydrates: 35-40 grams

- Dietary Fiber: 4-6 grams

- Sugars: 15-20 grams

Egg-in-the-Hole:

Prep Time: 5 minutes
Cook Time: 5 minutes
Servings: 1

Ingredients:

- 1 slice of bread (whole wheat or your choice)

- 1 egg

- 1 tablespoon butter

- Salt and pepper, to taste

Instructions:

1. Use a cookie cutter or the rim of a glass to cut a hole in the center of the bread slice.

2. Heat the butter in a skillet over medium heat until melted and sizzling.

3. Place the bread slice in the skillet and crack the egg into the hole in the center.

4. Season the egg with salt and pepper to taste.

5. Cook for 2-3 minutes, until the bottom of the bread is golden brown and crispy.

6. Carefully flip the bread and egg over using a spatula.

7. Continue cooking for another 2-3 minutes, or until the egg is cooked to your desired doneness.

8. Remove from the skillet and serve hot.

9. Enjoy this classic and comforting egg-in-the-hole for breakfast or brunch!

Nutritional Values (Approximate, per serving):

- Calories: 250-300 kcal

- Protein: 10-12 grams

- Fat: 15-18 grams

- Saturated Fat: 7-9 grams

- Carbohydrates: 15-20 grams

- Dietary Fiber: 1-2 grams

- Sugars: 2-3 grams

Skillet-Baked Pancake:

Prep Time: 10 minutes
Cook Time: 20 minutes
Servings: 4

Ingredients:

- 1 cup all-purpose flour

- 1 tablespoon sugar

- 1/2 teaspoon baking powder

- 1/4 teaspoon baking soda

- 1/4 teaspoon salt

- 2 large eggs

- 1 cup buttermilk

- 2 tablespoons unsalted butter, melted

- 1 teaspoon vanilla extract

- Powdered sugar, for dusting (optional)

- Maple syrup, for serving

Instructions:

1. Preheat your oven to 425°F (220°C).

2. In a mixing bowl, whisk together the flour, sugar, baking powder, baking soda, and salt.

3. In another bowl, beat the eggs, then whisk in the buttermilk, melted butter, and vanilla extract until well combined.

4. Pour the wet ingredients into the dry ingredients and stir until just combined. Do not overmix; it's okay if the batter is slightly lumpy.

5. Heat a cast-iron skillet over medium heat and add a little butter or oil to grease the bottom.

6. Once the skillet is hot, pour the pancake batter into the skillet and spread it evenly.

7. Transfer the skillet to the preheated oven and bake for 15-20 minutes, or until the pancake is puffed up and golden brown around the edges.

8. Remove from the oven and let cool for a few minutes.

9. Dust with powdered sugar if desired, slice into wedges, and serve warm with maple syrup.

Nutritional Values (Approximate, per serving):

- Calories: 200-250 kcal

- Protein: 6-8 grams

- Fat: 8-10 grams

- Saturated Fat: 4-6 grams

- Carbohydrates: 25-30 grams

- Dietary Fiber: 1-2 grams

- Sugars: 5-7 grams

Strawberry–Cream Cheese Stuffed French Toast:

Prep	**Time:**	15	minutes
Cook	**Time:**	10	minutes

Servings: 2

Ingredients:

- 4 slices of thick bread (such as brioche or challah)
- 1/4 cup cream cheese, softened
- 1/4 cup sliced strawberries
- 2 large eggs
- 1/4 cup milk (dairy or plant-based)
- 1/2 teaspoon vanilla extract
- 1/2 teaspoon ground cinnamon
- Butter or oil, for cooking
- Maple syrup, for serving

Instructions:

1. Spread cream cheese on two slices of bread. Top with sliced strawberries and cover with the remaining slices of bread to make sandwiches.

2. In a shallow dish, whisk together the eggs, milk, vanilla extract, and ground cinnamon.

3. Heat a skillet or griddle over medium heat and add a little butter or oil to grease the surface.

4. Dip each sandwich into the egg mixture, coating both sides evenly.

5. Place the dipped sandwiches in the skillet and cook for 3-4 minutes on each side, or until golden brown and cooked through.

6. Remove from the skillet and serve immediately with maple syrup.

Nutritional Values (Approximate, per serving):

- Calories: 350-400 kcal
- Protein: 12-15 grams
- Fat: 15-18 grams

- Saturated Fat: 7-9 grams

- Carbohydrates: 40-45 grams

- Dietary Fiber: 2-3 grams

- Sugars: 15-20 grams

Summer Vegetable Omelet:

Prep Time: 10 minutes
Cook Time: 10 minutes
Servings: 2

Ingredients:r

- 4 large eggs

- 2 tablespoons milk (dairy or plant-based)

- Salt and pepper, to taste

- 1 tablespoon olive oil

- 1/2 cup diced bell peppers

- 1/2 cup diced zucchini

- 1/2 cup diced tomatoes

- 1/4 cup chopped fresh basil

- 1/4 cup shredded cheese (such as cheddar or mozzarella)

Instructions:

1. In a bowl, whisk together the eggs, milk, salt, and pepper until well combined.

2. Heat olive oil in a skillet over medium heat.

3. Add diced bell peppers and zucchini to the skillet and sauté for 2-3 minutes, until slightly softened.

4. Pour the egg mixture into the skillet, tilting the pan to distribute the eggs evenly.

5. Cook the omelet for 2-3 minutes, lifting the edges with a spatula to let the uncooked eggs flow underneath.

6. Once the eggs are mostly set, sprinkle diced tomatoes, chopped fresh basil, and shredded cheese over one half of the omelet.

7. Carefully fold the other half of the omelet over the filling.

8. Cook for another 1-2 minutes, or until the cheese is melted and the omelet is cooked through.

9. Slide the omelet onto a plate, cut in half, and serve hot.

Nutritional Values (Approximate, per serving):

- Calories: 250-300 kcal

- Protein: 15-18 grams

- Fat: 18-20 grams

- Saturated Fat: 5-7 grams

- Carbohydrates: 6-8 grams

- Dietary Fiber: 1-2 grams

- Sugars: 4-6 grams

Cheesy Scrambled Eggs with Fresh Herbs:

Prep Time: 5 minutes
Cook Time: 5 minutes
Servings: 2

Ingredients:

- 4 large eggs

- 1/4 cup shredded cheddar cheese

- 1 tablespoon chopped fresh herbs (such as parsley, chives, or basil)

- Salt and pepper, to taste

- 1 tablespoon butter

Instructions:

1. Crack the eggs into a bowl and beat them lightly with a fork. Stir in the shredded cheddar cheese and chopped fresh herbs. Season with salt and pepper to taste.

2. Heat butter in a non-stick skillet over medium heat until melted and hot.

3. Pour the egg mixture into the skillet and let it cook undisturbed for a few seconds until the edges start to set.

4. Using a spatula, gently push the cooked edges toward the center of the skillet, allowing the uncooked eggs to flow to the edges.

5. Continue cooking and gently stirring until the eggs are softly set and slightly creamy.

6. Remove the skillet from the heat and transfer the scrambled eggs to a serving plate.

7. Garnish with additional fresh herbs if desired and serve hot.

Nutritional Values (Approximate, per serving):

- Calories: 200-250 kcal
- Protein: 14-16 grams
- Fat: 15-18 grams
- Saturated Fat: 7-9 grams
- Carbohydrates: 1-2 grams
- Dietary Fiber: 0 grams
- Sugars: 0 grams

Egg and Veggie Muffins:

Prep **Time:** 10 minutes
Cook **Time:** 20 minutes
Servings: 6

Ingredients:

- 6 large eggs
- 1/4 cup milk (dairy or plant-based)
- 1/2 cup diced bell peppers
- 1/2 cup diced tomatoes
- 1/4 cup chopped spinach
- 1/4 cup shredded cheddar cheese
- Salt and pepper, to taste

Instructions:

1. Preheat your oven to 350°F (175°C). Grease a muffin tin or line with paper liners.

2. In a bowl, whisk together the eggs and milk until well combined. Season with salt and pepper to taste.

3. Divide the diced bell peppers, tomatoes, chopped spinach, and shredded cheddar cheese evenly among the muffin cups.

4. Pour the egg mixture over the vegetables and cheese, filling each muffin cup about two-thirds full.

5. Bake in the preheated oven for 15-20 minutes, or until the egg muffins are set and lightly golden on top.

6. Remove from the oven and let cool for a few minutes before serving.

7. Enjoy these delicious and nutritious egg and veggie muffins for breakfast or as a snack.

Nutritional Values (Approximate, per serving):

- Calories: 100-150 kcal
- Protein: 8-10 grams
- Fat: 6-8 grams
- Saturated Fat: 3-5 grams

- Carbohydrates: 4-6 grams

- Dietary Fiber: 1-2 grams

- Sugars: 2-3 grams

Curried Egg Pita Pockets:

Prep Time: 10 minutes
Cook Time: 10 minutes
Servings: 2

Ingredients:

- 4 large eggs

- 1/4 cup Greek yogurt

- 1 teaspoon curry powder

- 1/4 cup diced cucumber

- 1/4 cup diced tomato

- 2 whole wheat pita pockets, halved

- Salt and pepper, to taste

- Fresh cilantro leaves, for garnish

Instructions:

1. Hard boil the eggs, then peel and chop them into small pieces.

2. In a bowl, mix together the chopped eggs, Greek yogurt, and curry powder until well combined. Season with salt and pepper to taste.

3. Gently fold in the diced cucumber and tomato.

4. Warm the whole wheat pita pockets in a toaster or oven.

5. Fill each pita pocket half with the curried egg salad mixture.

6. Garnish with fresh cilantro leaves.

7. Serve immediately and enjoy these flavorful curried egg pita pockets!

Nutritional Values (Approximate, per serving):

- Calories: 250-300 kcal

- Protein: 14-16 grams

- Fat: 10-12 grams

- Saturated Fat: 3-5 grams

- Carbohydrates: 25-30 grams

- Dietary Fiber: 4-6 grams

- Sugars: 3-5 grams

CHAPTER FOUR:

LUNCH

Grilled Lemon Herb Chicken Salad:

Prep Time: 20 minutes
Cook Time: 15 minutes
Servings: 4

Ingredients:

- 4 boneless, skinless chicken breasts
- 2 tablespoons olive oil
- 2 tablespoons fresh lemon juice
- 2 cloves garlic, minced
- 1 teaspoon dried oregano
- 1 teaspoon dried thyme
- Salt and pepper, to taste
- 6 cups mixed salad greens
- 1 cup cherry tomatoes, halved
- 1 cucumber, sliced
- 1/4 cup red onion, thinly sliced
- 1/4 cup feta cheese, crumbled

Instructions:

1. In a small bowl, whisk together olive oil, lemon juice, minced garlic, dried oregano, dried thyme, salt, and pepper to create the marinade.

2. Place the chicken breasts in a shallow dish and pour the marinade over them. Ensure the chicken is well coated. Let marinate for at least 15 minutes.

3. Preheat the grill to medium-high heat. Remove the chicken from the marinade and discard any excess marinade.

4. Grill the chicken for 6-7 minutes on each side, or until cooked through and no longer pink in the center. Remove from the grill and let rest for a few minutes before slicing.

5. In a large bowl, combine the mixed salad greens, cherry tomatoes, sliced cucumber, and thinly sliced red onion.

6. Divide the salad mixture onto serving plates. Top each salad with sliced grilled chicken breast.

7. Sprinkle crumbled feta cheese over the salads.

8. Serve immediately and enjoy this flavorful Grilled Lemon Herb Chicken Salad!

Nutritional Values (Approximate, per serving):

- Calories: 250-300 kcal

- Protein: 25-30 grams

- Fat: 10-12 grams

- Saturated Fat: 3-5 grams

- Carbohydrates: 10-12 grams

- Dietary Fiber: 2-3 grams

- Sugars: 2-3 grams

Vegetable Quinoa Stir-Fry:

Prep Time: 10 minutes
Cook Time: 20 minutes
Servings: 4

Ingredients:

- 1 cup quinoa, rinsed
- 2 cups water or low-sodium vegetable broth
- 2 tablespoons olive oil
- 2 cloves garlic, minced
- 1 onion, diced
- 2 carrots, sliced
- 1 bell pepper, sliced
- 1 cup broccoli florets
- 1 cup snap peas
- 1/4 cup low-sodium soy sauce
- 1 tablespoon sesame oil
- 1 tablespoon rice vinegar
- 1 teaspoon grated ginger
- Sesame seeds, for garnish (optional)
- Green onions, chopped, for garnish (optional)

Instructions:

1. In a medium saucepan, combine quinoa and water or vegetable broth. Bring to a boil, then reduce heat to low, cover, and simmer for 15-20 minutes, or until quinoa is cooked and liquid is absorbed. Fluff with a fork and set aside.

2. In a large skillet or wok, heat olive oil over medium-high heat. Add minced garlic and diced onion, and cook until softened and fragrant.

3. Add sliced carrots, bell pepper, broccoli florets, and snap peas to the skillet. Stir-fry for 5-7 minutes, or until vegetables are tender-crisp.

4. In a small bowl, whisk together low-sodium soy sauce, sesame oil, rice vinegar, and grated ginger to make the stir-fry sauce.

5. Add cooked quinoa to the skillet with the vegetables. Pour the stir-fry sauce over the quinoa and vegetables, and toss to combine.

6. Cook for an additional 2-3 minutes, or until everything is heated through and well coated in the sauce.

7. Remove from heat and garnish with sesame seeds and chopped green onions, if desired.

8. Serve hot and enjoy this nutritious and delicious Vegetable Quinoa Stir-Fry!

Nutritional Values (Approximate, per serving):

- Calories: 250-300 kcal
- Protein: 8-10 grams
- Fat: 8-10 grams
- Saturated Fat: 1-2 grams
- Carbohydrates: 35-40 grams
- Dietary Fiber: 5-7 grams
- Sugars: 5-7 grams

Salmon and Avocado Wrap:

Prep **Time:** 10 minutes
Cook **Time:** 10 minutes
Servings: 2

Ingredients:

- 2 whole wheat wraps or tortillas
- 2 salmon fillets
- 1 avocado, sliced
- 1 cup mixed salad greens
- 1/4 cup cherry tomatoes, halved
- 2 tablespoons Greek yogurt or sour cream
- 1 tablespoon lemon juice
- Salt and pepper, to taste

Instructions:

1. Season salmon fillets with salt, pepper, and lemon juice. Grill or pan-sear salmon until cooked through, about 4-5 minutes per side.
2. Warm whole wheat wraps or tortillas according to package **Instructions**.
3. In a small bowl, mash avocado with a fork and season with salt and pepper.
4. Spread mashed avocado onto each wrap or tortilla.
5. Top with mixed salad greens and cherry tomatoes.
6. Place grilled salmon fillets on top of the vegetables.
7. Drizzle Greek yogurt or sour cream over the salmon.
8. Roll up the wraps or tortillas tightly, and slice in half if desired.
9. Serve immediately and enjoy these delicious Salmon and Avocado Wraps!

Nutritional Values (Approximate, per serving):

- Calories: 350-400 kcal
- Protein: 25-30 grams
- Fat: 15-18 grams

- Saturated Fat: 3-5 grams

- Carbohydrates: 25-30 grams

- Dietary Fiber: 5-7 grams

- Sugars: 2-3 grams

Turkey and Veggie Lettuce Wraps:

Prep Time: 15 minutes
Cook Time: 15 minutes
Servings: 4

Ingredients:

- 1 lb lean ground turkey

- 1 tablespoon olive oil

- 1 onion, diced

- 2 cloves garlic, minced

- 1 bell pepper (red or green), diced

- 1 cup shredded carrots

- 1 cup water chestnuts, drained and chopped

- 1/4 cup low-sodium hoisin sauce

- 2 tablespoons low-sodium soy sauce

- 1 teaspoon sesame oil

- 1 head iceberg or butter lettuce, leaves separated

Instructions:

1. Heat olive oil in a large skillet over medium heat. Add diced onion and minced garlic, and sauté until fragrant.

2. Add lean ground turkey to the skillet and cook until browned, breaking it up with a spoon as it cooks.

3. Stir in diced bell pepper, shredded carrots, and chopped water chestnuts. Cook for an additional 3-4 minutes, or until vegetables are tender.

4. In a small bowl, whisk together low-sodium hoisin sauce, low-sodium soy sauce, and sesame oil. Pour the sauce over the turkey and vegetable mixture in the skillet.

5. Stir everything together until well combined and heated through.

6. To serve, spoon the turkey and vegetable mixture onto individual lettuce leaves.

7. Roll up the lettuce leaves to create wraps, securing them with toothpicks if needed.

8. Serve immediately and enjoy these flavorful and nutritious Turkey and Veggie Lettuce Wraps!

Nutritional Values (Approximate, per serving):

- Calories: 200-250 kcal
- Protein: 20-25 grams
- Fat: 8-10 grams
- Saturated Fat: 2-3 grams
- Carbohydrates: 10-12 grams
- Dietary Fiber: 2-3 grams
- Sugars: 4-6 grams

Mediterranean Chickpea Salad:

Prep Time: 15 minutes
Cook Time: 0 minutes
Servings: 4

Ingredients:

- 2 cans (15 oz each) chickpeas, drained and rinsed

- 1 cucumber, diced

- 1 bell pepper (red or green), diced

- 1 cup cherry tomatoes, halved

- 1/4 cup red onion, thinly sliced

- 1/4 cup Kalamata olives, sliced

- 1/4 cup crumbled feta cheese

- 2 tablespoons chopped fresh parsley

- 2 tablespoons extra virgin olive oil

- 2 tablespoons lemon juice

- 1 teaspoon dried oregano

- Salt and pepper, to taste

Instructions:

1. In a large bowl, combine chickpeas, diced cucumber, diced bell pepper, halved cherry tomatoes, thinly sliced red onion, sliced Kalamata olives, crumbled feta cheese, and chopped fresh parsley.

2. In a small bowl, whisk together extra virgin olive oil, lemon juice, dried oregano, salt, and pepper to make the dressing.

3. Pour the dressing over the chickpea salad and toss until everything is well coated.

4. Taste and adjust seasoning if needed.

5. Serve immediately or refrigerate for later.

6. Enjoy this refreshing and nutritious Mediterranean Chickpea Salad!

Nutritional Values (Approximate, per serving):

- Calories: 250-300 kcal

- Protein: 10-12 grams

- Fat: 12-15 grams

- Saturated Fat: 3-5 grams

- Carbohydrates: 30-35 grams

- Dietary Fiber: 8-10 grams

- Sugars: 5-7 grams

Sesame Ginger Tofu Stir-Fry:

Prep Time: 15 minutes
Cook Time: 15 minutes
Servings: 4

Ingredients:

- 1 block (14 oz) extra firm tofu, pressed and cubed
- 2 tablespoons low-sodium soy sauce
- 1 tablespoon sesame oil
- 2 cloves garlic, minced
- 1 tablespoon grated ginger
- 1 bell pepper, sliced
- 1 cup broccoli florets
- 1 cup sliced carrots
- 1 cup snap peas
- 2 tablespoons hoisin sauce
- 1 tablespoon rice vinegar
- 1 teaspoon cornstarch
- 2 tablespoons water
- Cooked brown rice, for serving
- Sesame seeds, for garnish (optional)
- Green onions, chopped, for garnish (optional)

Instructions:

1. In a bowl, toss cubed tofu with low-sodium soy sauce and sesame oil. Let marinate for 10-15 minutes.

2. Heat a large skillet or wok over medium-high heat. Add marinated tofu and cook until browned and crispy on all sides. Remove from skillet and set aside.

3. In the same skillet, add minced garlic and grated ginger. Cook until fragrant.

4. Add sliced bell pepper, broccoli florets, sliced carrots, and snap peas to the skillet. Stir-fry until vegetables are tender-crisp.

5. In a small bowl, whisk together hoisin sauce, rice vinegar, cornstarch, and water to make the sauce.

6. Pour the sauce over the stir-fried vegetables in the skillet. Stir until sauce thickens.

7. Add cooked tofu back to the skillet and toss until everything is well coated in the sauce.

8. Serve sesame ginger tofu stir-fry over cooked brown rice.

9. Garnish with sesame seeds and chopped green onions, if desired.

10. Enjoy this flavorful and healthy sesame ginger tofu stir-fry!

Nutritional Values (Approximate, per serving):

- Calories: 300-350 kcal

- Protein: 15-18 grams

- Fat: 12-15 grams

- Saturated Fat: 2-3 grams

- Carbohydrates: 35-40 grams

- Dietary Fiber: 8-10 grams

- Sugars: 10-12 grams

Caprese Quinoa Salad:

Prep Time: 15 minutes
Cook Time: 15 minutes
Servings: 4

Ingredients:

- 1 cup quinoa, rinsed
- 2 cups water or low-sodium vegetable broth
- 2 cups cherry tomatoes, halved
- 1 cup fresh mozzarella balls, halved
- 1/4 cup fresh basil leaves, chopped
- 2 tablespoons extra virgin olive oil
- 1 tablespoon balsamic vinegar
- Salt and pepper, to taste

Instructions:

1. In a medium saucepan, combine quinoa and water or vegetable broth. Bring to a boil, then reduce heat to low, cover, and simmer for 15-20 minutes, or until quinoa is cooked and liquid is absorbed. Fluff with a fork and let cool.

2. In a large bowl, combine cooked quinoa, halved cherry tomatoes, halved fresh mozzarella balls, and chopped fresh basil leaves.

3. In a small bowl, whisk together extra virgin olive oil, balsamic vinegar, salt, and pepper to make the dressing.

4. Pour the dressing over the quinoa salad and toss until everything is well coated.

5. Taste and adjust seasoning if needed.

6. Serve immediately or refrigerate for later.

7. Enjoy this refreshing and flavorful Caprese Quinoa Salad!

Nutritional Values (Approximate, per serving):

- Calories: 250-300 kcal
- Protein: 10-12 grams
- Fat: 12-15 grams

- Saturated Fat: 4-6 grams

- Carbohydrates: 25-30 grams

- Dietary Fiber: 3-5 grams

- Sugars: 3-5 grams

Veggie and Hummus Wrap:

Prep Time: 10 minutes
Cook Time: 0 minutes
Servings: 2

Ingredients:

- 2 whole wheat wraps or tortillas

- 1/2 cup hummus

- 1 cup mixed salad greens

- 1/2 cup shredded carrots

- 1/2 cup sliced cucumber

- 1/2 cup sliced bell pepper

- 1/4 cup sliced red onion

Instructions:

1. Lay out whole wheat wraps or tortillas on a clean work surface.

2. Spread hummus evenly over each wrap or tortilla.

3. Top with mixed salad greens, shredded carrots, sliced cucumber, sliced bell pepper, and sliced red onion.

4. Roll up the wraps or tortillas tightly, tucking in the sides as you go.

5. Slice the wraps in half if desired.

6. Serve immediately and enjoy these delicious Veggie and Hummus Wraps!

Nutritional Values (Approximate, per serving):

- Calories: 250-300 kcal

- Protein: 8-10 grams

- Fat: 10-12 grams

- Saturated Fat: 1-2 grams

- Carbohydrates: 30-35 grams

- Dietary Fiber: 6-8 grams

- Sugars: 2-3 grams

Greek Yogurt Chicken Salad:

Prep Time: 15 minutes
Cook Time: 15 minutes
Servings: 4

Ingredients:

- 2 cups cooked chicken breast, shredded or diced

- 1/2 cup Greek yogurt

- 1/4 cup diced celery

- 1/4 cup diced red onion

- 1/4 cup halved grapes

- 1/4 cup chopped walnuts

- 1 tablespoon lemon juice

- 1 tablespoon Dijon mustard

- Salt and pepper, to taste

- Lettuce leaves, for serving

Instructions:

1. In a large bowl, combine cooked chicken breast, Greek yogurt, diced celery, diced red onion, halved grapes, and chopped walnuts.

2. Add lemon juice and Dijon mustard to the bowl, and toss everything together until well combined.

3. Season with salt and pepper to taste, adjusting as needed.

4. Serve the Greek yogurt chicken salad on lettuce leaves as wraps or on top of a bed of mixed greens.

5. Enjoy this creamy and flavorful Greek Yogurt Chicken Salad!

Nutritional Values (Approximate, per serving):

- Calories: 200-250 kcal

- Protein: 20-25 grams

- Fat: 8-10 grams

- Saturated Fat: 1-2 grams

- Carbohydrates: 10-12 grams

- Dietary Fiber: 2-3 grams

- Sugars: 5-7 grams

Lentil and Vegetable Soup:

| **Prep** | **Time:** | 15 | minutes |
| **Cook** | **Time:** | 30 | minutes |

Servings: 4

Ingredients:

- 1 cup dry lentils, rinsed

- 4 cups low-sodium vegetable broth

- 1 onion, diced

- 2 carrots, diced

- 2 celery stalks, diced

- 2 cloves garlic, minced

- 1 can (14 oz) diced tomatoes

- 1 teaspoon dried thyme

- 1 teaspoon dried oregano

- Salt and pepper, to taste

- Fresh parsley, chopped, for garnish

Instructions:

1. In a large pot, combine rinsed lentils and low-sodium vegetable broth. Bring to a boil, then reduce heat to low, cover, and simmer for 15 minutes.

2. Add diced onion, diced carrots, diced celery, minced garlic, diced tomatoes, dried thyme, and dried oregano to the pot with the lentils.

3. Continue to simmer for an additional 15-20 minutes, or until lentils and vegetables are tender.

4. Season with salt and pepper to taste, adjusting as needed.

5. Ladle the lentil and vegetable soup into bowls, and garnish with chopped fresh parsley.

6. Serve hot and enjoy this hearty and nutritious Lentil and Vegetable Soup!

Nutritional Values (Approximate, per serving):

- Calories: 250-300 kcal

- Protein: 15-18 grams

- Fat: 2-4 grams

- Saturated Fat: 0-1 gram

- Carbohydrates: 45-50 grams

- Dietary Fiber: 15-18 grams

- Sugars: 6-8 grams

Cauliflower Fried Rice:

Prep   **Time:**   15   minutes

Cook   **Time:**   15   minutes

Servings: 4

Ingredients:

- 1 head cauliflower, riced (about 4 cups cauliflower rice)
- 2 tablespoons sesame oil
- 2 cloves garlic, minced
- 1 onion, diced
- 2 carrots, diced
- 1 cup frozen peas, thawed
- 2 eggs, lightly beaten
- 3 tablespoons low-sodium soy sauce
- 2 green onions, chopped
- Salt and pepper, to taste

Instructions:

1. In a large skillet or wok, heat sesame oil over medium heat.
2. Add minced garlic and diced onion to the skillet, and sauté until fragrant.
3. Add diced carrots to the skillet and cook until slightly tender.
4. Stir in riced cauliflower and thawed peas, and cook until cauliflower is tender, stirring occasionally.
5. Push the cauliflower mixture to one side of the skillet, and pour beaten eggs into the other side. Scramble the eggs until cooked through.
6. Once the eggs are cooked, mix them into the cauliflower mixture in the skillet.
7. Drizzle low-sodium soy sauce over the cauliflower fried rice, and toss everything together until well combined.
8. Season with salt and pepper to taste, adjusting as needed.
9. Garnish with chopped green onions before serving.
10. Enjoy this delicious and nutritious Cauliflower Fried Rice!

Nutritional Values (Approximate, per serving):

- Calories: 150-200 kcal

- Protein: 6-8 grams

- Fat: 8-10 grams

- Saturated Fat: 1-2 grams

- Carbohydrates: 15-20 grams

- Dietary Fiber: 5-7 grams

- Sugars: 5-7 grams

Shrimp and Avocado Salad:

| **Prep** | **Time:** | 15 | minutes |
| **Cook** | **Time:** | 5 | minutes |

Servings: 4

Ingredients:

- 1 lb shrimp, peeled and deveined

- 2 avocados, diced

- 1 cup cherry tomatoes, halved

- 1/4 cup red onion, thinly sliced

- 1/4 cup chopped fresh cilantro

- 1 tablespoon olive oil

- 1 tablespoon lime juice

- Salt and pepper, to taste

Instructions:

1. In a large skillet, heat olive oil over medium-high heat.

2. Add peeled and deveined shrimp to the skillet, and cook until pink and opaque, about 2-3 minutes per side. Remove from heat and let cool.

3. In a large bowl, combine diced avocados, halved cherry tomatoes, thinly sliced red onion, and chopped fresh cilantro.

4. Add cooked shrimp to the bowl with the avocado mixture.

5. Drizzle lime juice over the salad, and toss everything together until well combined.

6. Season with salt and pepper to taste, adjusting as needed.

7. Serve immediately and enjoy this fresh and flavorful Shrimp and Avocado Salad!

Nutritional Values (Approximate, per serving):

- Calories: 200-250 kcal
- Protein: 20-25 grams
- Fat: 10-12 grams
- Saturated Fat: 1-2 grams
- Carbohydrates: 10-12 grams
- Dietary Fiber: 6-8 grams
- Sugars: 2-3 grams

Prep   **Time:**   10   minutes

Cook   **Time:**   0   minutes

Servings: 4

Ingredients:

- 2 cans (5 oz each) tuna, drained
- 1 can (15 oz) white beans, drained and rinsed
- 1 cucumber, diced
- 1 bell pepper, diced
- 1/4 cup red onion, finely chopped
- 2 tablespoons chopped fresh parsley
- 2 tablespoons extra virgin olive oil
- 1 tablespoon lemon juice
- Salt and pepper, to taste

Instructions:

1. In a large bowl, combine drained tuna, white beans, diced cucumber, diced bell pepper, finely chopped red onion, and chopped fresh parsley.
2. Drizzle extra virgin olive oil and lemon juice over the salad ingredients.
3. Season with salt and pepper to taste, adjusting as needed.
4. Toss everything together until well combined.
5. Serve immediately or refrigerate for later.
6. Enjoy this protein-packed and nutritious Tuna and White Bean Salad!

Nutritional Values (Approximate, per serving):

- Calories: 250-300 kcal
- Protein: 20-25 grams
- Fat: 10-12 grams
- Saturated Fat: 2-3 grams
- Carbohydrates: 15-20 grams

- Dietary Fiber: 5-7 grams

- Sugars: 2-3 grams

Roasted Vegetable Quiche:

Prep Time: 15 minutes
Cook Time: 40 minutes
Servings: 6

Ingredients:

- 1 store-bought or homemade pie crust

- 2 cups mixed roasted vegetables (such as bell peppers, zucchini, onions, and mushrooms), chopped

- 1 cup shredded cheese (such as cheddar or Swiss)

- 4 large eggs

- 1 cup milk

- Salt and pepper, to taste

Instructions:

1. Preheat the oven to 375°F (190°C).

2. Roll out the pie crust and press it into a pie dish, trimming any excess dough.

3. Spread the chopped roasted vegetables evenly over the bottom of the pie crust.

4. Sprinkle shredded cheese over the roasted vegetables.

5. In a separate bowl, whisk together eggs, milk, salt, and pepper until well combined.

6. Pour the egg mixture over the roasted vegetables and cheese in the pie crust.

7. Bake in the preheated oven for 35-40 minutes, or until the quiche is set and golden brown on top.

8. Let the quiche cool for a few minutes before slicing and serving.

9. Enjoy this flavorful and satisfying Roasted Vegetable Quiche for lunch or dinner!

Nutritional Values (Approximate, per serving):

- Calories: 300-350 kcal

- Protein: 12-15 grams

- Fat: 18-20 grams

- Saturated Fat: 6-8 grams

- Carbohydrates: 20-25 grams

- Dietary Fiber: 2-3 grams

- Sugars: 2-3 grams

Soba Noodle Salad with Peanut Sauce:

Prep Time: 15 minutes
Cook Time: 5 minutes
Servings: 4

Ingredients:

- 8 oz soba noodles

- 1 cup shredded cabbage

- 1 carrot, julienned

- 1/2 red bell pepper, thinly sliced

- 2 green onions, thinly sliced

- 1/4 cup chopped cilantro

- 1/4 cup chopped roasted peanuts

- Sesame seeds, for garnish (optional)

Peanut Sauce:

- 1/4 cup creamy peanut butter

- 2 tablespoons soy sauce

- 1 tablespoon rice vinegar

- 1 tablespoon honey or maple syrup

- 1 tablespoon sesame oil

- 1 clove garlic, minced

- 1 teaspoon grated ginger

- 2-4 tablespoons water, to thin

Instructions:

1. Cook soba noodles according to package **Instructions**. Drain and rinse under cold water.

2. In a large bowl, combine cooked soba noodles, shredded cabbage, julienned carrot, thinly sliced red bell pepper, thinly sliced green onions, and chopped cilantro.

3. In a small bowl, whisk together creamy peanut butter, soy sauce, rice vinegar, honey or maple syrup, sesame oil, minced garlic, and grated ginger to make the peanut sauce. Add water gradually to thin the sauce to your desired consistency.

4. Pour the peanut sauce over the soba noodle salad and toss until everything is well coated.

5. Garnish with chopped roasted peanuts and sesame seeds, if desired.

6. Serve immediately or refrigerate for later.

7. Enjoy this flavorful and satisfying Soba Noodle Salad with Peanut Sauce!

Nutritional Values (Approximate, per serving):

- Calories: 300-350 kcal

- Protein: 8-10 grams

- Fat: 12-15 grams

- Saturated Fat: 2-3 grams

- Carbohydrates: 40-45 grams

- Dietary Fiber: 6-8 grams

- Sugars: 6-8 grams

CHAPTER FIVE:

DINNER

Grilled Lemon Herb Chicken Breast with Steamed Vegetables:

Prep Time: 15 minutes

Cook Time: 20 minutes

Servings: 4

Ingredients:

- 4 boneless, skinless chicken breasts
- 2 tablespoons olive oil
- 2 tablespoons fresh lemon juice
- 2 cloves garlic, minced
- 1 teaspoon dried thyme
- 1 teaspoon dried rosemary
- Salt and pepper to taste
- Assorted vegetables for steaming (such as broccoli, carrots, and cauliflower)

Instructions:

1. **Prepare the Marinade:** In a bowl, mix together olive oil, fresh lemon juice, minced garlic, dried thyme, dried rosemary, salt, and pepper.

2. **Marinate the Chicken:** Place chicken breasts in a shallow dish and pour the marinade over them, ensuring they are well coated. Let marinate for at least 30 minutes.

3. **Preheat the Grill:** Preheat grill to medium-high heat.

4. **Grill the Chicken:** Grill chicken breasts for about 6-7 minutes on each side or until cooked through.

5. **Steam the Vegetables:** While chicken is grilling, steam vegetables until tender yet crisp.

6. **Serve:** Serve grilled lemon herb chicken breast alongside steamed vegetables.

Nutritional Values (Approximate, per serving):

- Calories: 250 kcal

- Protein: 30 grams

- Fat: 12 grams

- Saturated Fat: 2 grams

- Carbohydrates: 8 grams

- Dietary Fiber: 3 grams

- Sugars: 3 grams

Baked Salmon with Dill Sauce and Roasted Asparagus:

Prep Time: 10 minutes

Cook Time: 15 minutes

Servings: 4

Ingredients:

- 4 salmon fillets
- 2 tablespoons olive oil
- Salt and pepper to taste
- 1 bunch asparagus, trimmed
- 2 tablespoons chopped fresh dill
- 1 tablespoon Dijon mustard
- 1 tablespoon honey
- 1 tablespoon lemon juice
- 1/4 cup plain Greek yogurt

Instructions:

1. **Preheat the Oven:** Preheat oven to 400°F (200°C). Line a baking sheet with parchment paper.

2. **Prepare the Salmon:** Place salmon fillets on the prepared baking sheet. Drizzle with olive oil and season with salt and pepper.

3. **Prepare the Asparagus:** Arrange trimmed asparagus around the salmon fillets on the baking sheet. Drizzle with a little olive oil and season with salt and pepper.

4. **Bake:** Bake in the preheated oven for about 12-15 minutes, or until salmon is cooked through and flakes easily with a fork.

5. **Prepare the Dill Sauce:** In a small bowl, mix together chopped fresh dill, Dijon mustard, honey, lemon juice, and Greek yogurt to make the dill sauce.

6. **Serve:** Serve baked salmon with roasted asparagus and drizzle with dill sauce.

Nutritional Values (Approximate, per serving):

- Calories: 300 kcal

- Protein: 25 grams

- Fat: 15 grams

- Saturated Fat: 3 grams

- Carbohydrates: 10 grams

- Dietary Fiber: 3 grams

- Sugars: 5 grams

Prep **Time:** 15 minutes

Cook **Time:** 20 minutes

Servings: 4

Ingredients:

- 1 lb shrimp, peeled and deveined
- 2 tablespoons olive oil
- 4 cloves garlic, minced
- 2 tablespoons lemon juice
- Zest of 1 lemon
- Salt and pepper to taste
- 1 cup quinoa
- 2 cups vegetable broth
- 1/2 cup chopped fresh parsley

Instructions:

1. **Cook Quinoa:** Rinse quinoa under cold water. In a saucepan, bring vegetable broth to a boil. Add quinoa, reduce heat to low, cover, and simmer for 15 minutes or until liquid is absorbed.

2. **Prepare Shrimp:** In a skillet, heat olive oil over medium heat. Add minced garlic and cook until fragrant, about 1 minute. Add shrimp, lemon juice, lemon zest, salt, and pepper. Cook shrimp until pink and cooked through, about 3-4 minutes per side.

3. **Fluff Quinoa:** Once quinoa is cooked, fluff it with a fork and stir in chopped fresh parsley.

4. **Serve:** Serve lemon garlic shrimp over quinoa pilaf. Enjoy!

Nutritional Values (Approximate, per serving):

- Calories: 350 kcal
- Protein: 25 grams
- Fat: 10 grams

- Saturated Fat: 1 gram

- Carbohydrates: 40 grams

- Dietary Fiber: 5 grams

- Sugars: 1 gram

Turkey Meatballs in Marinara Sauce served over Whole Wheat Pasta:

Prep Time: 20 minutes

Cook Time: 25 minutes

Servings: 4

Ingredients:

- 1 lb lean ground turkey

- 1/2 cup breadcrumbs

- 1/4 cup grated Parmesan cheese

- 1 egg

- 2 cloves garlic, minced

- 2 tablespoons chopped fresh parsley

- Salt and pepper to taste

- 2 cups marinara sauce

- 8 oz whole wheat spaghetti, cooked according to package **Instructions**

- Chopped fresh basil for garnish

Instructions:

1. **Prepare Meatballs:** In a bowl, combine ground turkey, breadcrumbs, Parmesan cheese, egg, minced garlic, chopped parsley, salt, and pepper. Mix until well combined. Form mixture into meatballs.

2. **Cook Meatballs:** In a skillet, heat olive oil over medium heat. Add meatballs and cook until browned on all sides and cooked through, about 10-12 minutes.

3. **Warm Marinara Sauce:** In a separate saucepan, heat marinara sauce over medium heat until warmed through.

4. **Serve:** Serve turkey meatballs over cooked whole wheat spaghetti. Top with warm marinara sauce and garnish with chopped fresh basil. Enjoy!

Nutritional Values (Approximate, per serving):

- Calories: 400 kcal

- Protein: 30 grams

- Fat: 10 grams

- Saturated Fat: 2 grams

- Carbohydrates: 45 grams

- Dietary Fiber: 8 grams

- Sugars: 6 grams

Roasted Chicken Thighs with Sweet Potatoes and Green Beans:

Prep **Time:** 15 minutes

Cook **Time:** 40 minutes

Servings: 4

Ingredients:

- 4 chicken thighs, bone-in and skin-on
- 2 sweet potatoes, peeled and diced
- 1 lb green beans, trimmed
- 2 tablespoons olive oil
- 2 cloves garlic, minced
- 1 teaspoon paprika
- 1 teaspoon dried thyme
- Salt and pepper to taste
- Fresh lemon wedges for serving

Instructions:

1. **Preheat Oven:** Preheat oven to 400°F (200°C).
2. **Prepare Chicken and Vegetables:** In a large bowl, toss chicken thighs, diced sweet potatoes, and green beans with olive oil, minced garlic, paprika, dried thyme, salt, and pepper until well coated.
3. **Roast:** Arrange chicken thighs, sweet potatoes, and green beans on a baking sheet lined with parchment paper. Roast in the preheated oven for 35-40 minutes or until chicken is cooked through and vegetables are tender.
4. **Serve:** Serve roasted chicken thighs with sweet potatoes and green beans. Squeeze fresh lemon juice over the dish before serving. Enjoy!

Nutritional Values (Approximate, per serving):

- Calories: 380 kcal
- Protein: 25 grams
- Fat: 15 grams

- Saturated Fat: 3 grams

- Carbohydrates: 30 grams

- Dietary Fiber: 7 grams

- Sugars: 8 grams

Baked Cod with Herbed Cauliflower Rice:

Prep Time: 15 minutes

Cook Time: 25 minutes

Servings: 4

Ingredients:

- 4 cod fillets

- 1 head cauliflower, grated or processed into rice

- 2 tablespoons olive oil

- 2 cloves garlic, minced

- 2 tablespoons chopped fresh parsley

- 1 tablespoon chopped fresh dill

- Salt and pepper to taste

- Lemon wedges for serving

Instructions:

1. **Preheat Oven:** Preheat the oven to 400°F (200°C).

2. **Prepare Cod:** Place cod fillets on a baking sheet lined with parchment paper. Drizzle with olive oil and season with salt and pepper.

3. **Bake:** Bake cod in the preheated oven for 15-20 minutes or until fish is cooked through and flakes easily with a fork.

4. **Prepare Cauliflower Rice:** In a skillet, heat olive oil over medium heat. Add minced garlic and cook until fragrant, about 1 minute. Add cauliflower rice and cook for 5-7 minutes, stirring occasionally, until cauliflower is tender. Stir in chopped parsley and dill. Season with salt and pepper to taste.

5. **Serve:** Serve baked cod with herbed cauliflower rice. Garnish with lemon wedges. Enjoy!

Nutritional Values (Approximate, per serving):

- Calories: 250 kcal

- Protein: 25 grams

- Fat: 10 grams

- Saturated Fat: 1 gram

- Carbohydrates: 10 grams

- Dietary Fiber: 5 grams

- Sugars: 3 grams

Vegetable Stir-Fry with Tofu served over Brown Rice:

Prep Time: 20 minutes

Cook Time: 15 minutes

Servings: 4

Ingredients:

- 1 block extra-firm tofu, pressed and cubed
- 2 cups mixed vegetables (bell peppers, broccoli, carrots, snow peas, etc.), sliced
- 2 tablespoons soy sauce
- 1 tablespoon sesame oil
- 2 cloves garlic, minced
- 1 tablespoon minced ginger
- Cooked brown rice for serving
- Chopped green onions and sesame seeds for garnish

Instructions:

1. **Prepare Tofu:** In a skillet, heat sesame oil over medium-high heat. Add cubed tofu and cook until golden brown on all sides, about 8-10 minutes. Remove tofu from skillet and set aside.

2. **Stir-Fry Vegetables:** In the same skillet, add a little more sesame oil if needed. Add minced garlic and ginger, and stir-fry for about 1 minute. Add mixed vegetables and stir-fry until crisp-tender, about 5-7 minutes.

3. **Combine:** Return cooked tofu to the skillet with the vegetables. Add soy sauce and toss to combine.

4. **Serve:** Serve vegetable stir-fry with tofu over cooked brown rice. Garnish with chopped green onions and sesame seeds. Enjoy!

Nutritional Values (Approximate, per serving):

- Calories: 300 kcal
- Protein: 15 grams
- Fat: 10 grams

- Saturated Fat: 1 gram

- Carbohydrates: 35 grams

- Dietary Fiber: 8 grams

- Sugars: 5 grams

Eggplant Parmesan with Mixed Green Salad:

Prep Time: 20 minutes

Cook Time: 45 minutes

Servings: 4

Ingredients: For Eggplant Parmesan:

- 2 large eggplants, sliced into 1/2-inch rounds

- 2 cups breadcrumbs

- 1 cup grated Parmesan cheese

- 2 eggs, beaten

- 2 cups marinara sauce

- 1 cup shredded mozzarella cheese

- Fresh basil leaves for garnish

- Salt and pepper to taste

- Olive oil for frying

For Mixed Green Salad:

- 4 cups mixed greens (lettuce, spinach, arugula, etc.)

- 1 cup cherry tomatoes, halved

- 1/2 cucumber, sliced

- 1/4 red onion, thinly sliced

- 1/4 cup balsamic vinaigrette dressing

Instructions:

1. **Preheat Oven:** Preheat the oven to 375°F (190°C).

2. **Bread Eggplant:** In one shallow bowl, place beaten eggs. In another shallow bowl, mix breadcrumbs, grated Parmesan cheese, salt, and pepper. Dip each eggplant slice into the beaten eggs, then coat with breadcrumb mixture.

3. **Fry Eggplant:** In a large skillet, heat olive oil over medium heat. Fry breaded eggplant slices until golden brown on both sides, about 2-3 minutes per side. Place fried eggplant slices on a paper towel-lined plate to drain excess oil.

4. **Assemble Eggplant Parmesan:** In a baking dish, spread a thin layer of marinara sauce. Arrange a layer of fried eggplant slices on top. Spoon more marinara sauce over the eggplant, then sprinkle with shredded mozzarella cheese. Repeat layers until all ingredients are used, finishing with a layer of cheese on top.

5. **Bake:** Cover the baking dish with foil and bake in the preheated oven for 30 minutes. Remove foil and bake for an additional 15 minutes, or until cheese is bubbly and golden brown.

6. **Prepare Salad:** In a large bowl, toss mixed greens, cherry tomatoes, cucumber, and red onion with balsamic vinaigrette dressing until evenly coated.

7. **Serve:** Serve Eggplant Parmesan hot, garnished with fresh basil leaves, alongside mixed green salad. Enjoy!

Nutritional Values (Approximate, per serving):

- Calories: 450 kcal

- Protein: 20 grams

- Fat: 20 grams

- Saturated Fat: 7 grams

- Carbohydrates: 45 grams

- Dietary Fiber: 10 grams

- Sugars: 15 grams

Beef Stir-Fry with Broccoli and Bell Peppers:

Prep Time: 15 minutes

Cook Time: 15 minutes

Servings: 4

Ingredients:

- 1 lb beef sirloin, thinly sliced
- 2 cups broccoli florets
- 1 red bell pepper, sliced
- 1 yellow bell pepper, sliced
- 1 onion, sliced
- 2 cloves garlic, minced
- 1 tablespoon ginger, minced
- 3 tablespoons soy sauce
- 2 tablespoons oyster sauce
- 1 tablespoon sesame oil
- 1 tablespoon vegetable oil
- Salt and pepper to taste
- Cooked rice, for serving

Instructions:

1. In a bowl, marinate the sliced beef with soy sauce, minced garlic, and minced ginger. Let it marinate for at least 15 minutes.
2. Heat vegetable oil in a large skillet or wok over medium-high heat.
3. Add the marinated beef slices to the skillet and stir-fry until browned and cooked through, about 2-3 minutes. Remove from the skillet and set aside.
4. In the same skillet, add a bit more oil if needed. Add the sliced onions and bell peppers, and stir-fry for 2-3 minutes until they start to soften.
5. Add the broccoli florets to the skillet and continue to stir-fry for another 2-3 minutes until the vegetables are tender-crisp.

6. Return the cooked beef to the skillet. Add soy sauce, oyster sauce, and sesame oil. Stir-fry everything together for an additional 1-2 minutes to combine and heat through.

7. Season with salt and pepper to taste.

8. Serve the beef stir-fry with broccoli and bell peppers hot over cooked rice.

9. Enjoy this flavorful and nutritious beef stir-fry as a satisfying dinner option!

Nutritional Values (Approximate, per serving):

- Calories: 300-350 kcal

- Protein: 25-30 grams

- Fat: 10-12 grams

- Saturated Fat: 3-4 grams

- Carbohydrates: 20-25 grams

- Dietary Fiber: 4-6 grams

- Sugars: 6-8 grams

Prep **Time:** 15 minutes

Cook **Time:** 45 minutes

Servings: 6

Ingredients:

- 1 cup dried lentils, rinsed and drained
- 1 onion, chopped
- 2 carrots, diced
- 2 stalks celery, diced
- 3 cloves garlic, minced
- 1 can (14 oz) diced tomatoes
- 4 cups vegetable broth
- 2 cups water
- 1 teaspoon dried thyme
- 1 teaspoon dried oregano
- Salt and pepper to taste
- Fresh parsley, chopped, for garnish
- Whole grain bread rolls, for serving

Instructions:

1. In a large pot, heat some oil over medium heat. Add the chopped onion, carrots, and celery, and sauté until softened, about 5-7 minutes.

2. Add the minced garlic and sauté for another minute until fragrant.

3. Stir in the rinsed lentils, diced tomatoes, vegetable broth, water, dried thyme, and dried oregano. Bring the soup to a boil.

4. Once boiling, reduce the heat to low, cover, and let the soup simmer for about 30-40 minutes, or until the lentils are tender.

5. Season the soup with salt and pepper to taste.

6. Serve the lentil soup hot, garnished with chopped fresh parsley, and accompanied by whole grain bread rolls.

Nutritional Values (Approximate, per serving):

- Calories: 200-250 kcal
- Protein: 10-12 grams
- Fat: 2-3 grams
- Saturated Fat: 0.5-1 gram
- Carbohydrates: 35-40 grams
- Dietary Fiber: 10-12 grams
- Sugars: 6-8 grams

Prep **Time**: 20 minutes

Cook **Time**: 30 minutes

Servings: 4

Ingredients:

- 1 cup brown rice
- 2 cups water
- 1 tablespoon olive oil
- 1 onion, chopped
- 2 cloves garlic, minced
- 1 tablespoon ginger, grated
- 1 tablespoon curry powder
- 1 teaspoon ground cumin
- 1 teaspoon ground coriander
- 1 can (14 oz) coconut milk
- 2 cups mixed vegetables (such as bell peppers, carrots, broccoli, and peas)
- Salt and pepper to taste
- Fresh cilantro, chopped, for garnish

Instructions:

1. In a saucepan, combine the brown rice and water. Bring to a boil, then reduce the heat to low, cover, and simmer for about 20-25 minutes, or until the rice is tender and the water is absorbed.

2. In a large skillet, heat the olive oil over medium heat. Add the chopped onion and sauté until softened, about 5 minutes.

3. Add the minced garlic, grated ginger, curry powder, ground cumin, and ground coriander to the skillet. Cook for another minute until fragrant.

4. Pour in the coconut milk and stir to combine. Bring the mixture to a simmer.

5. Add the mixed vegetables to the skillet and simmer for about 10-15 minutes, or until the vegetables are tender.

6. Season the vegetable curry with salt and pepper to taste.

7. Serve the vegetable curry hot over cooked brown rice, garnished with fresh chopped cilantro.

Nutritional Values (Approximate, per serving):

- Calories: 300-350 kcal

- Protein: 6-8 grams

- Fat: 15-18 grams

- Saturated Fat: 10-12 grams

- Carbohydrates: 35-40 grams

- Dietary Fiber: 6-8 grams

- Sugars: 2-4 grams

Grilled Portobello Mushrooms with Balsamic Glaze and Couscous:

Prep Time: 10 minutes

Cook Time: 15 minutes

Servings: 2

Ingredients:

- 2 large portobello mushrooms
- 2 tablespoons balsamic vinegar
- 1 tablespoon olive oil
- 2 cloves garlic, minced
- Salt and pepper, to taste
- 1 cup couscous
- 1 1/4 cups vegetable broth or water
- Fresh parsley, chopped, for garnish

Instructions:

1. Preheat the grill to medium-high heat.
2. Clean the portobello mushrooms and remove the stems.
3. In a small bowl, whisk together the balsamic vinegar, olive oil, minced garlic, salt, and pepper to make the marinade.
4. Brush the marinade over both sides of the portobello mushrooms.
5. Place the mushrooms on the grill and cook for about 5-7 minutes on each side, or until tender and grill marks appear.
6. While the mushrooms are grilling, prepare the couscous according to the package **Instructions**, using vegetable broth or water for added flavor.
7. Serve the grilled portobello mushrooms over a bed of couscous, drizzled with any remaining balsamic glaze from the marinade.
8. Garnish with chopped fresh parsley and enjoy!

Nutritional Values (Approximate, per serving):

- Calories: 250-300 kcal

- Protein: 8-10 grams

- Fat: 5-7 grams

- Saturated Fat: 1 gram

- Carbohydrates: 45-50 grams

- Dietary Fiber: 5-7 grams

- Sugars: 3-5 grams

Baked Tilapia with Lemon and Garlic, served with Roasted Brussels Sprouts:

Prep Time: 10 minutes

Cook Time: 20 minutes

Servings: 2

Ingredients:

- 2 tilapia fillets

- 1 lemon, thinly sliced

- 2 cloves garlic, minced

- 2 tablespoons olive oil

- Salt and pepper, to taste

- 1 pound Brussels sprouts, trimmed and halved

- 1 tablespoon balsamic vinegar (optional)

- Fresh parsley, chopped, for garnish

Instructions:

1. Preheat the oven to 400°F (200°C).

2. Place the tilapia fillets on a baking sheet lined with parchment paper. Season with salt, pepper, and minced garlic. Top each fillet with thinly sliced lemon.

3. Drizzle the tilapia with olive oil and bake in the preheated oven for about 15-20 minutes, or until the fish is cooked through and flakes easily with a fork.

4. While the tilapia is baking, toss the halved Brussels sprouts with olive oil, salt, and pepper on another baking sheet.

5. Roast the Brussels sprouts in the oven alongside the tilapia for about 20-25 minutes, or until golden brown and tender.

6. If desired, drizzle the roasted Brussels sprouts with balsamic vinegar for extra flavor.

7. Serve the baked tilapia and roasted Brussels sprouts together, garnished with chopped fresh parsley.

8. Enjoy this nutritious and flavorful meal!

Nutritional Values (Approximate, per serving):

- Calories: 300-350 kcal

- Protein: 30-35 grams

- Fat: 12-15 grams

- Saturated Fat: 2-3 grams

- Carbohydrates: 20-25 grams

- Dietary Fiber: 8-10 grams

- Sugars: 4-6 grams

| **Prep** | **Time:** | 15 | minutes |
| **Cook** | **Time:** | 30 | minutes |

Servings: 4

Ingredients:

- 1 eggplant, diced
- 2 zucchinis, diced
- 1 yellow bell pepper, diced
- 1 red bell pepper, diced
- 1 onion, diced
- 2 cloves garlic, minced
- 2 tomatoes, diced
- 2 tablespoons tomato paste
- 1 tablespoon olive oil
- 1 teaspoon dried thyme
- 1 teaspoon dried oregano
- Salt and pepper, to taste
- 1 cup quinoa
- 2 cups vegetable broth or water
- Fresh basil, chopped, for garnish

Instructions:

1. In a large skillet, heat the olive oil over medium heat. Add the diced onion and minced garlic, and sauté until softened, about 2-3 minutes.

2. Add the diced eggplant, zucchini, bell peppers, and tomatoes to the skillet. Cook, stirring occasionally, until the vegetables are tender, about 10-15 minutes.

3. Stir in the tomato paste, dried thyme, dried oregano, salt, and pepper. Cook for an additional 5 minutes, allowing the flavors to meld together.

4. While the ratatouille is cooking, rinse the quinoa under cold water. In a separate pot, combine the quinoa and vegetable broth or water. Bring to a boil, then reduce

the heat to low, cover, and simmer for 15-20 minutes, or until the quinoa is cooked and the liquid is absorbed.

5. Once the quinoa is cooked, fluff it with a fork and divide it among serving plates.

6. Spoon the ratatouille over the quinoa, garnish with chopped fresh basil, and serve hot.

7. Enjoy this hearty and flavorful ratatouille served over quinoa!

Nutritional Values (Approximate, per serving):

- Calories: 250-300 kcal

- Protein: 8-10 grams

- Fat: 5-7 grams

- Saturated Fat: 1 gram

- Carbohydrates: 45-50 grams

- Dietary Fiber: 8-10 grams

- Sugars: 6-8 grams

Chicken and Vegetable Skewers with Brown Rice Pilaf:

Prep Time: 20 minutes

Cook Time: 20 minutes

Servings: 4

Ingredients:

- 2 chicken breasts, cut into cubes
- 1 red bell pepper, cut into chunks
- 1 yellow bell pepper, cut into chunks
- 1 red onion, cut into chunks
- 8 cherry tomatoes
- 8 wooden skewers, soaked in water for 30 minutes
- 2 tablespoons olive oil
- 2 cloves garlic, minced
- 1 teaspoon dried thyme
- 1 teaspoon paprika
- Salt and pepper, to taste
- 1 cup brown rice
- 2 cups chicken broth or water
- Fresh parsley, chopped, for garnish

Instructions:

1. Preheat the grill or grill pan to medium-high heat.

2. Thread the chicken cubes, bell pepper chunks, red onion chunks, and cherry tomatoes onto the soaked wooden skewers, alternating between ingredients.

3. In a small bowl, whisk together the olive oil, minced garlic, dried thyme, paprika, salt, and pepper to make the marinade. Brush the marinade over the skewers.

4. Grill the skewers for 10-12 minutes, turning occasionally, or until the chicken is cooked through and the vegetables are tender and slightly charred.

5. While the skewers are grilling, rinse the brown rice under cold water. In a separate pot, combine the brown rice and chicken broth or water. Bring to a boil, then reduce the heat to low, cover, and simmer for 15-20 minutes, or until the rice is cooked and the liquid is absorbed.

6. Once the rice is cooked, fluff it with a fork and divide it among serving plates.

7. Serve the grilled chicken and vegetable skewers over the brown rice, garnished with chopped fresh parsley.

8. Enjoy these delicious and colorful chicken skewers with brown rice pilaf!

Nutritional Values (Approximate, per serving):

- Calories: 350-400 kcal

- Protein: 25-30 grams

- Fat: 8-10 grams

- Saturated Fat: 1-2 grams

- Carbohydrates: 45-50 grams

- Dietary Fiber: 6-8 grams

- Sugars: 4-6 grams

CHAPTER SIX:

Hearty and Nourishing Soup Recipes

French Onion Soup:

Prep Time: 10 minutes

Cook Time: 1 hour

Servings: 4

Ingredients:

- 4 large onions, thinly sliced
- 2 tablespoons butter
- 2 tablespoons olive oil
- 4 cups beef broth
- 1 cup dry white wine
- 1 teaspoon Worcestershire sauce
- Salt and pepper, to taste
- 4 slices of toasted French bread
- 1 cup shredded Gruyere or Swiss cheese

Instructions:

1. In a large pot, melt the butter with the olive oil over medium heat.

2. Add the sliced onions to the pot and cook, stirring occasionally, until they are caramelized and golden brown, about 30-40 minutes.

3. Pour in the beef broth, white wine, and Worcestershire sauce. Season with salt and pepper to taste.

4. Bring the soup to a simmer and let it cook for an additional 20-30 minutes to allow the flavors to meld.

5. Preheat the oven broiler. Ladle the hot soup into oven-safe bowls.

6. Top each bowl with a slice of toasted French bread and sprinkle with shredded Gruyere or Swiss cheese.

7. Place the bowls under the broiler until the cheese is melted and bubbly, about 2-3 minutes.

8. Carefully remove the bowls from the oven and serve hot.

9. Enjoy this comforting French Onion Soup!

Nutritional Values (Approximate, per serving):

- Calories: 300-350 kcal

- Protein: 10-12 grams

- Fat: 15-18 grams

- Saturated Fat: 7-9 grams

- Carbohydrates: 20-25 grams

- Dietary Fiber: 2-3 grams

- Sugars: 6-8 grams

Cream of Watercress Soup:

Prep   **Time:**   15   minutes

Cook   **Time:**   25   minutes

Servings: 4

Ingredients:

- 1 bunch of watercress, stems removed
- 1 onion, chopped
- 2 cloves garlic, minced
- 2 tablespoons butter
- 2 tablespoons all-purpose flour
- 4 cups vegetable broth
- 1 cup heavy cream
- Salt and pepper, to taste
- Fresh watercress leaves, for garnish (optional)

Instructions:

1. In a large pot, melt the butter over medium heat. Add the chopped onion and minced garlic, and sauté until softened, about 5 minutes.

2. Add the watercress to the pot and cook until wilted, about 3-4 minutes.

3. Sprinkle the flour over the vegetables and stir to combine, cooking for an additional 2 minutes.

4. Gradually pour in the vegetable broth, stirring constantly to prevent lumps from forming.

5. Bring the soup to a simmer and let it cook for about 15 minutes, allowing the flavors to meld.

6. Use an immersion blender to puree the soup until smooth. Alternatively, carefully transfer the soup to a blender and blend until smooth, then return it to the pot.

7. Stir in the heavy cream and season with salt and pepper to taste.

8. Continue to cook the soup for another 5 minutes, stirring occasionally.

9. Ladle the soup into bowls and garnish with fresh watercress leaves, if desired.

10. Serve hot and enjoy this creamy and flavorful Cream of Watercress Soup!

Nutritional Values (Approximate, per serving):

- Calories: 250-300 kcal

- Protein: 4-6 grams

- Fat: 20-25 grams

- Saturated Fat: 12-15 grams

- Carbohydrates: 15-20 grams

- Dietary Fiber: 2-3 grams

- Sugars: 3-5 grams

Curried Cauliflower Soup:

Prep Time: 15 minutes

Cook Time: 30 minutes

Servings: 4

Ingredients:

- 1 large cauliflower, chopped into florets

- 1 onion, chopped

- 2 cloves garlic, minced

- 2 tablespoons olive oil

- 2 teaspoons curry powder

- 4 cups vegetable broth

- 1 cup coconut milk

- Salt and pepper, to taste

- Fresh cilantro, for garnish (optional)

Instructions:

1. In a large pot, heat the olive oil over medium heat. Add the chopped onion and minced garlic, and sauté until softened, about 5 minutes.

2. Stir in the curry powder and cook for an additional 2 minutes, until fragrant.

3. Add the cauliflower florets to the pot and pour in the vegetable broth.

4. Bring the mixture to a boil, then reduce the heat to low and let it simmer for about 20 minutes, or until the cauliflower is tender.

5. Use an immersion blender to puree the soup until smooth. Alternatively, carefully transfer the soup to a blender and blend until smooth, then return it to the pot.

6. Stir in the coconut milk and season with salt and pepper to taste.

7. Continue to cook the soup for another 5 minutes, stirring occasionally.

8. Ladle the soup into bowls and garnish with fresh cilantro, if desired.

9. Serve hot and enjoy this delicious and aromatic Curried Cauliflower Soup!

Nutritional Values (Approximate, per serving):

- Calories: 200-250 kcal

- Protein: 4-6 grams

- Fat: 15-18 grams

- Saturated Fat: 10-12 grams

- Carbohydrates: 15-20 grams

- Dietary Fiber: 4-6 grams

- Sugars: 5-7 grams

Prep Time: 15 minutes

Cook Time: 35 minutes

Servings: 4

Ingredients:

- 2 large red bell peppers
- 1 medium eggplant, diced
- 1 onion, chopped
- 2 cloves garlic, minced
- 2 tablespoons olive oil
- 4 cups vegetable broth
- 1 teaspoon dried thyme
- Salt and pepper, to taste
- Fresh basil leaves, for garnish (optional)

Instructions:

1. Preheat the oven to 400°F (200°C). Line a baking sheet with parchment paper.

2. Place the whole red bell peppers on the prepared baking sheet and roast in the preheated oven for 20-25 minutes, or until the skins are charred and blistered, turning occasionally.

3. Remove the bell peppers from the oven and transfer them to a bowl. Cover the bowl with plastic wrap and let the peppers steam for about 10 minutes.

4. Once cooled, peel off the skins of the roasted bell peppers, remove the seeds and stems, and roughly chop the flesh.

5. In a large pot, heat the olive oil over medium heat. Add the chopped onion and minced garlic, and sauté until softened, about 5 minutes.

6. Add the diced eggplant to the pot and cook for another 5 minutes, until slightly softened.

7. Stir in the roasted red peppers, vegetable broth, and dried thyme. Season with salt and pepper to taste.

8. Bring the soup to a simmer, then reduce the heat to low and let it cook for about 15 minutes, allowing the flavors to meld.

9. Use an immersion blender to puree the soup until smooth. Alternatively, carefully transfer the soup to a blender and blend until smooth, then return it to the pot.

10. Continue to cook the soup for another 5 minutes, stirring occasionally.

11. Ladle the soup into bowls and garnish with fresh basil leaves, if desired.

12. Serve hot and enjoy this rich and flavorful Roasted Red Pepper and Eggplant Soup!

Nutritional Values (Approximate, per serving):

- Calories: 150-200 kcal

- Protein: 2-3 grams

- Fat: 8-10 grams

- Saturated Fat: 1-2 grams

- Carbohydrates: 15-20 grams

- Dietary Fiber: 4-6 grams

- Sugars: 8-10 grams

Prep **Time:** 15 minutes

Cook **Time:** 40 minutes

Servings: 6

Ingredients:

- 1 tablespoon olive oil

- 1 onion, chopped

- 2 carrots, peeled and sliced

- 2 celery stalks, sliced

- 2 cloves garlic, minced

- 6 cups chicken broth

- 2 cups diced cooked chicken breast

- 1 cup diced potatoes

- 1 cup diced tomatoes

- 1 cup frozen green peas

- 1 teaspoon dried thyme

- Salt and pepper, to taste

- Fresh parsley, for garnish (optional)

Instructions:

1. In a large pot, heat the olive oil over medium heat. Add the chopped onion, sliced carrots, and sliced celery, and sauté until softened, about 5 minutes.

2. Add the minced garlic to the pot and cook for an additional 2 minutes, until fragrant.

3. Pour in the chicken broth and bring the mixture to a simmer.

4. Add the diced chicken breast, diced potatoes, diced tomatoes, frozen green peas, and dried thyme to the pot.

5. Season the soup with salt and pepper to taste.

6. Let the soup simmer for about 25-30 minutes, or until the vegetables are tender and the flavors have melded.

7. Taste and adjust the seasoning if necessary.

8. Ladle the soup into bowls and garnish with fresh parsley, if desired.

9. Serve hot and enjoy this comforting Traditional Chicken-Vegetable Soup!

Nutritional Values (Approximate, per serving):

- Calories: 200-250 kcal

- Protein: 15-18 grams

- Fat: 5-7 grams

- Saturated Fat: 1-2 grams

- Carbohydrates: 15-20 grams

- Dietary Fiber: 4-6 grams

- Sugars: 4-6 grams

Prep   **Time:**   15   minutes

Cook   **Time:**   30   minutes

Servings: 4

Ingredients:

- 1 tablespoon olive oil
- 1 onion, chopped
- 2 carrots, diced
- 2 celery stalks, diced
- 2 cloves garlic, minced
- 1 lb (450g) ground turkey
- 1/2 cup bulgur wheat
- 6 cups chicken broth
- 1 teaspoon dried thyme
- Salt and pepper, to taste
- Fresh parsley, chopped, for garnish (optional)

Instructions:

1. In a large pot, heat the olive oil over medium heat. Add the chopped onion, diced carrots, and diced celery, and sauté until softened, about 5 minutes.

2. Add the minced garlic to the pot and cook for an additional 2 minutes, until fragrant.

3. Add the ground turkey to the pot and cook until browned, breaking it up with a spoon as it cooks.

4. Stir in the bulgur wheat, chicken broth, and dried thyme. Season with salt and pepper to taste.

5. Bring the soup to a simmer, then reduce the heat to low and let it cook for about 20-25 minutes, or until the bulgur is tender and the flavors have melded.

6. Taste and adjust the seasoning if necessary.

7. Ladle the soup into bowls and garnish with fresh parsley, if desired.

8. Serve hot and enjoy this hearty and nutritious Turkey-Bulgur Soup!

Nutritional Values (Approximate, per serving):

- Calories: 250-300 kcal

- Protein: 20-25 grams

- Fat: 10-12 grams

- Saturated Fat: 2-3 grams

- Carbohydrates: 15-20 grams

- Dietary Fiber: 4-6 grams

- Sugars: 4-6 grams

Ground Beef and Rice Soup:

Prep	**Time:**	15	minutes
Cook	**Time:**	30	minutes

Servings: 4

Ingredients:

- 1 tablespoon olive oil

- 1 onion, chopped

- 2 carrots, diced

- 2 celery stalks, diced

- 2 cloves garlic, minced

- 1 lb (450g) lean ground beef

- 1/2 cup long-grain white rice

- 6 cups beef broth

- 1 teaspoon dried thyme

- Salt and pepper, to taste

- Fresh parsley, chopped, for garnish (optional)

Instructions:

1. In a large pot, heat the olive oil over medium heat. Add the chopped onion, diced carrots, and diced celery, and sauté until softened, about 5 minutes.

2. Add the minced garlic to the pot and cook for an additional 2 minutes, until fragrant.

3. Add the lean ground beef to the pot and cook until browned, breaking it up with a spoon as it cooks.

4. Stir in the white rice, beef broth, and dried thyme. Season with salt and pepper to taste.

5. Bring the soup to a simmer, then reduce the heat to low and let it cook for about 20-25 minutes, or until the rice is tender and the flavors have melded.

6. Taste and adjust the seasoning if necessary.

7. Ladle the soup into bowls and garnish with fresh parsley, if desired.

8. Serve hot and enjoy this comforting Ground Beef and Rice Soup!

Nutritional Values (Approximate, per serving):

- Calories: 300-350 kcal
- Protein: 20-25 grams
- Fat: 15-18 grams
- Saturated Fat: 5-7 grams
- Carbohydrates: 20-25 grams
- Dietary Fiber: 2-3 grams
- Sugars: 2-3 grams

Prep Time: 15 minutes

Cook Time: 30 minutes

Servings: 4

Ingredients:

- 1 tablespoon olive oil
- 1 onion, diced
- 2 cloves garlic, minced
- 4 cups green cabbage, shredded
- 2 carrots, diced
- 2 celery stalks, diced
- 1 can (14 oz) diced tomatoes
- 4 cups vegetable broth
- 1 teaspoon dried thyme
- 1 teaspoon dried rosemary
- Salt and pepper, to taste
- Fresh parsley, chopped, for garnish (optional)

Instructions:

1. In a large pot, heat the olive oil over medium heat. Add the diced onion and minced garlic, and sauté until softened and fragrant, about 5 minutes.

2. Add the shredded cabbage, diced carrots, and diced celery to the pot. Cook, stirring occasionally, for about 5-7 minutes, until the vegetables begin to soften.

3. Stir in the diced tomatoes (with their juices), vegetable broth, dried thyme, and dried rosemary. Season with salt and pepper to taste.

4. Bring the stew to a simmer, then reduce the heat to low and let it cook for about 20-25 minutes, stirring occasionally, until the vegetables are tender and the flavors have melded.

5. Taste and adjust the seasoning if necessary.

6. Ladle the stew into bowls, garnish with chopped fresh parsley if desired, and serve hot.

7. Enjoy this comforting and flavorful Herbed Cabbage Stew!

Nutritional Values (Approximate, per serving):

- Calories: 150-200 kcal

- Protein: 4-6 grams

- Fat: 4-6 grams

- Saturated Fat: 1 gram

- Carbohydrates: 20-25 grams

- Dietary Fiber: 6-8 grams

- Sugars: 8-10 grams

Winter Chicken Stew:

Prep Time: 15 minutes

Cook Time: 45 minutes

Servings: 4

Ingredients:

- 1 tablespoon olive oil

- 1 onion, diced

- 2 cloves garlic, minced

- 2 carrots, diced

- 2 celery stalks, diced

- 1 lb (450g) boneless, skinless chicken breasts, diced

- 4 cups chicken broth

- 1 cup diced potatoes

- 1 cup diced butternut squash

- 1 teaspoon dried thyme

- 1 teaspoon dried rosemary

- Salt and pepper, to taste

- Fresh parsley, chopped, for garnish (optional)

Instructions:

1. In a large pot, heat the olive oil over medium heat. Add the diced onion and minced garlic, and sauté until softened and fragrant, about 5 minutes.

2. Add the diced carrots and diced celery to the pot. Cook, stirring occasionally, for about 5 minutes, until the vegetables begin to soften.

3. Add the diced chicken to the pot and cook until browned on all sides.

4. Stir in the chicken broth, diced potatoes, diced butternut squash, dried thyme, and dried rosemary. Season with salt and pepper to taste.

5. Bring the stew to a simmer, then reduce the heat to low and let it cook for about 30-35 minutes, stirring occasionally, until the chicken is cooked through and the vegetables are tender.

6. Taste and adjust the seasoning if necessary.

7. Ladle the stew into bowls, garnish with chopped fresh parsley if desired, and serve hot.

8. Enjoy this hearty and warming Winter Chicken Stew!

Nutritional Values (Approximate, per serving):

- Calories: 250-300 kcal

- Protein: 20-25 grams

- Fat: 6-8 grams

- Saturated Fat: 1-2 grams

- Carbohydrates: 20-25 grams

- Dietary Fiber: 4-6 grams

- Sugars: 4-6 grams

Prep	**Time**:	15	minutes
Cook	**Time**:	2 hours 30	minutes

Servings: 6

Ingredients:

- 2 lbs (900g) beef chuck roast, cut into cubes
- 2 tablespoons olive oil
- 1 onion, chopped
- 3 cloves garlic, minced
- 3 carrots, peeled and sliced
- 2 celery stalks, sliced
- 2 cups beef broth
- 1 cup red wine (optional)
- 2 tablespoons tomato paste
- 2 bay leaves
- 1 teaspoon dried thyme
- Salt and pepper, to taste
- 2 tablespoons all-purpose flour (optional, for thickening)
- Chopped fresh parsley, for garnish (optional)

Instructions:

1. Preheat the oven to 325°F (160°C).

2. In a large oven-safe pot or Dutch oven, heat the olive oil over medium-high heat. Add the beef cubes in batches and cook until browned on all sides. Remove the beef from the pot and set aside.

3. In the same pot, add the chopped onion and minced garlic. Cook until softened and fragrant, about 5 minutes.

4. Add the sliced carrots and celery to the pot and cook for another 5 minutes, stirring occasionally.

5. Return the browned beef cubes to the pot. Add the beef broth, red wine (if using), tomato paste, bay leaves, dried thyme, salt, and pepper. Stir to combine.

6. Cover the pot with a lid and transfer it to the preheated oven. Let the stew roast for 2 to 2 1/2 hours, or until the beef is tender and the flavors have melded.

7. If you prefer a thicker stew, you can make a slurry by mixing 2 tablespoons of flour with some water and stir it into the stew during the last 30 minutes of cooking.

8. Once the stew is done cooking, remove it from the oven. Taste and adjust the seasoning if necessary.

9. Discard the bay leaves and garnish the stew with chopped fresh parsley, if desired, before serving.

10. Serve hot and enjoy this comforting Roasted Beef Stew!

Nutritional Values (Approximate, per serving):

- Calories: 350-400 kcal

- Protein: 30-35 grams

- Fat: 20-25 grams

- Saturated Fat: 7-9 grams

- Carbohydrates: 10-15 grams

- Dietary Fiber: 2-4 grams

- Sugars: 3-5 grams

1. **Read Labels**: Always read the nutrition labels carefully to identify the sodium content per serving. Choose soups labeled as "low-sodium" or "reduced sodium" whenever possible.

2. **Choose Broth-Based Soups**: Opt for soups with a clear broth base rather than creamy or cheesy soups, as they tend to have lower sodium levels.

3. **Look for Unsalted Varieties**: Some brands offer unsalted or no-salt-added versions of their soups. These can be a good option for reducing sodium intake.

4. **Dilute with Water**: If you have a high-sodium soup, you can dilute it with water or low-sodium broth to reduce the sodium concentration per serving.

5. **Rinse Canned Beans**: If the soup contains canned beans, rinse them under cold water before adding them to the soup. This can help reduce the sodium content.

6. **Add Fresh Herbs and Spices**: Enhance the flavor of the soup with fresh herbs and spices instead of salt. Use ingredients like garlic, onions, basil, thyme, rosemary, and black pepper to add flavor without increasing sodium.

7. **Limit Added Salt**: If you need to add salt to your soup, do so sparingly. Taste the soup first and then add salt if necessary. You may find that you don't need as much salt when you enhance the flavor with other ingredients.

8. **Choose Vegetable-Based Soups**: Vegetable-based soups tend to have lower sodium levels compared to meat-based soups. Consider opting for vegetable soups or those with minimal meat content.

9. **Make Homemade Soups**: Consider making your own soups at home using fresh ingredients. This gives you full control over the sodium content and allows you to customize the flavor to your liking.

10. **Use Low-Sodium Broth**: When preparing homemade soups, use low-sodium or no-salt-added broth as the base. This helps control the overall sodium content of the soup.

Vibrant Salad Creations with Homemade Dressings

Leaf Lettuce and Carrot Salad with Balsamic Vinaigrette:

Prep Time: 10 minutes

Servings: 2

Ingredients:

- 4 cups leaf lettuce, torn into bite-sized pieces
- 1 large carrot, grated
- 2 tablespoons balsamic vinegar
- 1 tablespoon extra virgin olive oil
- 1 teaspoon honey
- Salt and pepper, to taste

Instructions:

1. In a large mixing bowl, combine the torn leaf lettuce and grated carrot.
2. In a small bowl, whisk together the balsamic vinegar, extra virgin olive oil, honey, salt, and pepper to make the vinaigrette.
3. Pour the vinaigrette over the lettuce and carrot mixture.
4. Toss the salad gently until the vegetables are evenly coated with the dressing.
5. Divide the salad into individual serving bowls.
6. Serve immediately and enjoy this refreshing Leaf Lettuce and Carrot Salad with Balsamic Vinaigrette!

Nutritional Values (Approximate, per serving):

- Calories: 70-90 kcal
- Protein: 1-2 grams
- Fat: 4-6 grams
- Saturated Fat: 0.5-1 gram
- Carbohydrates: 8-10 grams

- Dietary Fiber: 2-3 grams

- Sugars: 5-7 grams

Strawberry-Watercress Salad with Almond Dressing:

Prep Time: 15 minutes

Servings: 2

Ingredients:

- 4 cups watercress, washed and trimmed

- 1 cup fresh strawberries, sliced

- 2 tablespoons sliced almonds, toasted

- 2 tablespoons almond butter

- 2 tablespoons water

- 1 tablespoon lemon juice

- 1 teaspoon honey or maple syrup

- Salt and pepper, to taste

Instructions:

1. In a large mixing bowl, combine the watercress and sliced strawberries.

2. In a small bowl, whisk together the almond butter, water, lemon juice, honey or maple syrup, salt, and pepper to make the dressing.

3. Pour the almond dressing over the watercress and strawberry mixture.

4. Toss the salad gently until the greens and fruit are evenly coated with the dressing.

5. Divide the salad into individual serving plates.

6. Sprinkle the toasted sliced almonds over the top of each salad.

7. Serve immediately and enjoy this delightful Strawberry-Watercress Salad with Almond Dressing!

Nutritional Values (Approximate, per serving):

- Calories: 120-150 kcal
- Protein: 4-6 grams
- Fat: 8-10 grams
- Saturated Fat: 1-2 grams
- Carbohydrates: 10-12 grams
- Dietary Fiber: 4-5 grams
- Sugars: 6-8 grams

Cucumber-Dill Cabbage Salad with Lemon Dressing:

Prep Time: 15 minutes

Servings: 4

Ingredients:

- 4 cups shredded cabbage

- 1 cucumber, thinly sliced

- 2 tablespoons chopped fresh dill

- 2 tablespoons lemon juice

- 1 tablespoon extra virgin olive oil

- 1 teaspoon honey or maple syrup

- Salt and pepper, to taste

Instructions:

1. In a large mixing bowl, combine the shredded cabbage, sliced cucumber, and chopped fresh dill.

2. In a small bowl, whisk together the lemon juice, extra virgin olive oil, honey or maple syrup, salt, and pepper to make the dressing.

3. Pour the lemon dressing over the cabbage, cucumber, and dill mixture.

4. Toss the salad gently until the vegetables are evenly coated with the dressing.

5. Serve immediately or refrigerate for later.

6. Enjoy this refreshing Cucumber-Dill Cabbage Salad with Lemon Dressing as a side dish or light meal!

Nutritional Values (Approximate, per serving):

- Calories: 50-70 kcal

- Protein: 1-2 grams

- Fat: 3-5 grams

- Saturated Fat: 0.5-1 gram

- Carbohydrates: 6-8 grams

- Dietary Fiber: 2-3 grams

- Sugars: 3-4 grams

Leaf Lettuce and Asparagus Salad with Raspberries:

Prep Time: 20 minutes

Servings: 2

Ingredients:

- 4 cups torn leaf lettuce

- 1 cup asparagus spears, blanched and sliced

- 1/2 cup fresh raspberries

- 2 tablespoons sliced almonds, toasted

- 2 tablespoons balsamic vinegar

- 1 tablespoon extra virgin olive oil

- 1 teaspoon honey or maple syrup

- Salt and pepper, to taste

Instructions:

1. In a large mixing bowl, combine the torn leaf lettuce, blanched and sliced asparagus, fresh raspberries, and sliced almonds.

2. In a small bowl, whisk together the balsamic vinegar, extra virgin olive oil, honey or maple syrup, salt, and pepper to make the dressing.

3. Pour the balsamic dressing over the salad ingredients.

4. Toss the salad gently until the greens and asparagus are evenly coated with the dressing.

5. Divide the salad into individual serving plates.

6. Serve immediately and enjoy this vibrant Leaf Lettuce and Asparagus Salad with Raspberries!

Nutritional Values (Approximate, per serving):

- Calories: 120-150 kcal

- Protein: 4-6 grams

- Fat: 8-10 grams

- Saturated Fat: 1-2 grams

- Carbohydrates: 12-15 grams

- Dietary Fiber: 5-7 grams

- Sugars: 6-8 grams

Waldorf Salad:

Prep Time: 15 minutes

Servings: 4

Ingredients:

- 2 medium apples, cored and diced

- 1 cup seedless grapes, halved

- 1 cup celery, thinly sliced

- 1/2 cup walnuts, chopped

- 1/4 cup mayonnaise

- 2 tablespoons plain Greek yogurt

- 1 tablespoon lemon juice

- 1 tablespoon honey

- Salt and pepper, to taste

- Lettuce leaves, for serving (optional)

Instructions:

1. In a large mixing bowl, combine the diced apples, halved grapes, sliced celery, and chopped walnuts.

2. In a small bowl, whisk together the mayonnaise, Greek yogurt, lemon juice, honey, salt, and pepper to make the dressing.

3. Pour the dressing over the apple, grape, celery, and walnut mixture.

4. Toss the salad gently until all ingredients are evenly coated with the dressing.

5. Serve the Waldorf salad on a bed of lettuce leaves if desired.

6. Enjoy this classic Waldorf Salad as a refreshing side dish or light meal!

Nutritional Values (Approximate, per serving):

- Calories: 200-250 kcal

- Protein: 3-4 grams

- Fat: 14-18 grams

- Saturated Fat: 1-2 grams

- Carbohydrates: 20-25 grams

- Dietary Fiber: 3-4 grams

- Sugars: 15-20 grams

Asian Pear Salad:

Prep Time: 15 minutes

Servings: 4

Ingredients:

- 2 Asian pears, cored and thinly sliced
- 4 cups mixed salad greens
- 1/4 cup sliced almonds, toasted
- 1/4 cup crumbled feta cheese
- 2 tablespoons dried cranberries
- 2 tablespoons balsamic vinegar
- 1 tablespoon extra virgin olive oil
- 1 teaspoon honey
- Salt and pepper, to taste

Instructions:

1. In a large salad bowl, combine the sliced Asian pears, mixed salad greens, toasted sliced almonds, crumbled feta cheese, and dried cranberries.
2. In a small bowl, whisk together the balsamic vinegar, extra virgin olive oil, honey, salt, and pepper to make the dressing.
3. Pour the dressing over the salad ingredients.
4. Toss the salad gently until the greens and pears are evenly coated with the dressing.
5. Divide the salad into individual serving plates.
6. Serve immediately and enjoy this refreshing Asian Pear Salad!

Nutritional Values (Approximate, per serving):

- Calories: 150-200 kcal
- Protein: 3-4 grams
- Fat: 8-10 grams
- Saturated Fat: 2-3 grams

- Carbohydrates: 20-25 grams

- Dietary Fiber: 4-6 grams

- Sugars: 14-18 grams

Couscous Salad with Spicy Citrus Dressing:

Prep Time: 15 minutes

Cook Time: 10 minutes

Servings: 4

Ingredients:

- 1 cup couscous

- 1 1/4 cups vegetable broth or water

- 1/4 cup orange juice

- Zest of 1 orange

- 2 tablespoons lemon juice

- 1 tablespoon lime juice

- 2 tablespoons extra virgin olive oil

- 1 teaspoon honey

- 1/2 teaspoon ground cumin

- 1/4 teaspoon chili powder

- Salt and pepper, to taste

- 1/4 cup chopped fresh cilantro

- 1/4 cup chopped fresh mint

- 1/4 cup sliced almonds, toasted

- 1/4 cup dried cranberries

- 1/4 cup diced red bell pepper

- 1/4 cup diced cucumber

- 1/4 cup crumbled feta cheese (optional)

Instructions:

1. In a medium saucepan, bring the vegetable broth or water to a boil. Stir in the couscous, cover, and remove from heat. Let it sit for about 5 minutes, then fluff with a fork and transfer to a large mixing bowl to cool.

2. In a small bowl, whisk together the orange juice, orange zest, lemon juice, lime juice, extra virgin olive oil, honey, ground cumin, chili powder, salt, and pepper to make the dressing.

3. Pour the dressing over the cooled couscous and toss to coat.

4. Add the chopped cilantro, chopped mint, toasted sliced almonds, dried cranberries, diced red bell pepper, diced cucumber, and crumbled feta cheese (if using) to the couscous mixture.

5. Toss gently until all ingredients are well combined.

6. Serve the couscous salad immediately or refrigerate until ready to serve.

7. Enjoy this vibrant Couscous Salad with Spicy Citrus Dressing as a light and flavorful meal or side dish!

Nutritional Values (Approximate, per serving):

- Calories: 250-300 kcal

- Protein: 6-8 grams

- Fat: 8-10 grams

- Saturated Fat: 1-2 grams

- Carbohydrates: 40-45 grams

- Dietary Fiber: 4-6 grams

- Sugars: 6-8 grams

Prep **Time:** 15 minutes

Cook **Time:** 10 minutes

Servings: 4

Ingredients:

- 8 oz farfalle pasta (bowtie pasta)
- 1 cup cherry tomatoes, halved
- 1/2 cup diced red bell pepper
- 1/2 cup diced yellow bell pepper
- 1/2 cup diced green bell pepper
- 1/4 cup diced red onion
- 1/4 cup sliced black olives
- 1/4 cup crumbled feta cheese (optional)
- 2 tablespoons chopped fresh parsley
- 2 tablespoons chopped fresh basil
- 2 tablespoons extra virgin olive oil
- 1 tablespoon balsamic vinegar
- 1 clove garlic, minced
- Salt and pepper, to taste

Instructions:

1. Cook the farfalle pasta according to package **Instructions** until al dente. Drain and rinse under cold water to cool.

2. In a large mixing bowl, combine the cooked farfalle pasta, halved cherry tomatoes, diced red bell pepper, diced yellow bell pepper, diced green bell pepper, diced red onion, sliced black olives, crumbled feta cheese (if using), chopped parsley, and chopped basil.

3. In a small bowl, whisk together the extra virgin olive oil, balsamic vinegar, minced garlic, salt, and pepper to make the dressing.

4. Pour the dressing over the pasta salad and toss until all ingredients are well coated.

5. Serve the Farfalle Confetti Salad immediately or refrigerate until ready to serve.

6. Enjoy this colorful and flavorful pasta salad as a refreshing meal or side dish!

Nutritional Values (Approximate, per serving):

- Calories: 300-350 kcal

- Protein: 8-10 grams

- Fat: 10-12 grams

- Saturated Fat: 2-3 grams

- Carbohydrates: 45-50 grams

- Dietary Fiber: 4-6 grams

- Sugars: 4-6 grams

Prep   Time: 15   minutes

Cook   Time: 0   minutes

Servings: 4

Ingredients:

- 1 cup bulgur wheat
- 1 1/2 cups boiling water
- 2 cups chopped fresh parsley
- 1/2 cup chopped fresh mint
- 1/2 cup diced cucumber
- 1/2 cup diced tomato
- 1/4 cup finely chopped red onion
- 2 tablespoons extra virgin olive oil
- 2 tablespoons lemon juice
- Salt and pepper, to taste

Instructions:

1. Place the bulgur wheat in a heatproof bowl and pour the boiling water over it. Cover the bowl with a lid or plastic wrap and let it sit for about 15 minutes, or until the bulgur is tender and has absorbed all the water.

2. Fluff the cooked bulgur with a fork and let it cool to room temperature.

3. In a large mixing bowl, combine the cooked bulgur, chopped parsley, chopped mint, diced cucumber, diced tomato, and finely chopped red onion.

4. Drizzle the extra virgin olive oil and lemon juice over the salad ingredients.

5. Season with salt and pepper, to taste.

6. Toss the tabbouleh gently until all ingredients are well combined and evenly coated with the dressing.

7. Serve immediately or refrigerate until ready to serve.

8. Enjoy this fresh and flavorful Tabbouleh salad as a side dish or light meal!

Nutritional Values (Approximate, per serving):

- Calories: 150-200 kcal

- Protein: 4-6 grams

- Fat: 6-8 grams

- Saturated Fat: 1 gram

- Carbohydrates: 20-25 grams

- Dietary Fiber: 4-6 grams

- Sugars: 1-2 grams

Prep Time: 15 minutes

Cook Time: 10 minutes

Servings: 4

Ingredients:

- 1 lb flank steak, thinly sliced
- 2 tablespoons soy sauce
- 2 tablespoons hoisin sauce
- 1 tablespoon rice vinegar
- 1 tablespoon honey
- 1 tablespoon grated fresh ginger
- 2 cloves garlic, minced
- 2 tablespoons vegetable oil
- 4 cups mixed salad greens
- 1/2 cup shredded carrots
- 1/2 cup sliced cucumber
- 1/4 cup chopped green onions
- 2 tablespoons chopped fresh cilantro
- 1 tablespoon sesame seeds (optional)

Instructions:

1. In a small bowl, whisk together the soy sauce, hoisin sauce, rice vinegar, honey, grated ginger, and minced garlic to make the marinade.

2. Place the thinly sliced flank steak in a shallow dish and pour the marinade over it. Toss to coat the steak evenly. Let it marinate for at least 15 minutes.

3. Heat the vegetable oil in a skillet or grill pan over medium-high heat. Add the marinated flank steak and cook for about 3-4 minutes per side, or until cooked to your desired doneness. Remove from heat and let it rest for a few minutes before slicing.

4. In a large mixing bowl, combine the mixed salad greens, shredded carrots, sliced cucumber, chopped green onions, and chopped cilantro.

5. Arrange the salad mixture on serving plates or bowls.

6. Top the salad with the sliced ginger beef.

7. Sprinkle sesame seeds over the salad, if desired.

8. Serve immediately and enjoy this delicious and satisfying Ginger Beef Salad!

Nutritional Values (Approximate, per serving):

- Calories: 300-350 kcal

- Protein: 25-30 grams

- Fat: 15-18 grams

- Saturated Fat: 4-6 grams

- Carbohydrates: 15-20 grams

- Dietary Fiber: 2-4 grams

- Sugars: 8-10 grams

CHAPTER SEVEN:

Appetizers and Snacks

Roasted Onion Garlic Dip:

Prep Time: 10 minutes

Cook Time: 30 minutes

Servings: 6

Ingredients:

- 2 large onions, peeled and chopped
- 4 cloves garlic, minced
- 2 tablespoons olive oil
- 1 cup plain Greek yogurt
- 2 tablespoons lemon juice
- Salt and pepper to taste
- Chopped fresh parsley for garnish (optional)

Instructions:

1. Preheat the oven to 400°F (200°C).
2. In a baking dish, toss the chopped onions and minced garlic with olive oil until evenly coated.
3. Roast in the preheated oven for about 25-30 minutes or until the onions are caramelized and tender, stirring occasionally.
4. Remove from the oven and let cool slightly.
5. In a food processor, combine the roasted onions and garlic with Greek yogurt and lemon juice. Blend until smooth.
6. Season with salt and pepper to taste.
7. Transfer the dip to a serving bowl and garnish with chopped fresh parsley if desired.
8. Serve with vegetable sticks, pita chips, or crackers.
9. Enjoy your Roasted Onion Garlic Dip!

Nutritional Values (Approximate, per serving):

- Calories: 70-90 kcal

- Protein: 3-4 grams

- Fat: 4-6 grams

- Carbohydrates: 6-8 grams

- Dietary Fiber: 1-2 grams

- Sugars: 2-3 grams

Baba Ghanoush:

Prep Time: 15 minutes

Cook Time: 45 minutes

Servings: 4

Ingredients:

- 2 large eggplants

- 2 cloves garlic, minced

- 2 tablespoons tahini

- 2 tablespoons lemon juice

- 2 tablespoons extra virgin olive oil

- Salt to taste

- Chopped fresh parsley for garnish (optional)

- Paprika for garnish (optional)

Instructions:

1. Preheat the oven to 400°F (200°C).

2. Pierce the eggplants with a fork in several places and place them on a baking sheet lined with parchment paper.

3. Roast the eggplants in the preheated oven for about 45 minutes or until they are soft and collapse.

4. Remove the eggplants from the oven and let them cool slightly.

5. Peel the skin off the eggplants and discard.

6. In a food processor, combine the roasted eggplant flesh, minced garlic, tahini, lemon juice, and olive oil. Blend until smooth.

7. Season with salt to taste.

8. Transfer the Baba Ghanoush to a serving bowl and drizzle with a little extra olive oil.

9. Garnish with chopped fresh parsley and a sprinkle of paprika if desired.

10. Serve with pita bread, crackers, or vegetable sticks.

11. Enjoy your delicious Baba Ghanoush!

Nutritional Values (Approximate, per serving):

- Calories: 100-120 kcal

- Protein: 2-3 grams

- Fat: 7-9 grams

- Carbohydrates: 8-10 grams

- Dietary Fiber: 3-4 grams

- Sugars: 3-4 grams

| **Prep** | **Time**: | 10 | minutes |
| **Cook** | **Time**: | 0 | minutes |

Servings: 4

Ingredients:

- 1 cup plain Greek yogurt
- 1/2 cup grated cheese (such as cheddar or Parmesan)
- 1 tablespoon chopped fresh herbs (such as parsley, chives, or dill)
- 1 clove garlic, minced
- 1 tablespoon lemon juice
- Salt and pepper to taste

Instructions:

1. In a mixing bowl, combine the plain Greek yogurt, grated cheese, chopped fresh herbs, minced garlic, and lemon juice.
2. Stir until well combined.
3. Season with salt and pepper to taste.
4. Transfer the dip to a serving bowl.
5. Serve with vegetable sticks, pretzels, or crackers.
6. Enjoy your Cheese-Herb Dip!

Nutritional Values (Approximate, per serving):

- Calories: 70-90 kcal
- Protein: 8-10 grams
- Fat: 3-4 grams
- Carbohydrates: 2-3 grams
- Dietary Fiber: 0 grams
- Sugars: 1-2 grams

Spicy Kale Chips:

Prep Time: 10 minutes

Cook Time: 15 minutes

Servings: 4

Ingredients:

- 1 bunch kale, washed and dried
- 1 tablespoon olive oil
- 1 teaspoon paprika
- 1/2 teaspoon garlic powder
- 1/2 teaspoon chili powder
- Salt to taste

Instructions:

1. Preheat the oven to 325°F (160°C). Line a baking sheet with parchment paper.
2. Remove the stems from the kale leaves and tear the leaves into bite-sized pieces.
3. In a large bowl, toss the kale pieces with olive oil until evenly coated.
4. In a small bowl, mix together the paprika, garlic powder, chili powder, and salt.
5. Sprinkle the spice mixture over the kale and toss until the leaves are coated.
6. Arrange the kale pieces in a single layer on the prepared baking sheet.
7. Bake in the preheated oven for 12-15 minutes, or until the kale is crispy and slightly browned around the edges.
8. Remove from the oven and let cool slightly before serving.
9. Serve your Spicy Kale Chips as a healthy and flavorful snack.
10. Enjoy!

Nutritional Values (Approximate, per serving):

- Calories: 60-80 kcal
- Protein: 2-3 grams
- Fat: 3-4 grams
- Carbohydrates: 5-6 grams

- Dietary Fiber: 1-2 grams

- Sugars: 1-2 grams

Cinnamon Tortilla Chips:

Prep Time: 5 minutes

Cook Time: 10 minutes

Servings: 4

Ingredients:

- 4 large flour tortillas

- 2 tablespoons melted butter or coconut oil

- 2 tablespoons granulated sugar

- 1 teaspoon ground cinnamon

Instructions:

1. Preheat the oven to 350°F (175°C). Line a baking sheet with parchment paper.

2. Brush both sides of each tortilla with melted butter or coconut oil.

3. In a small bowl, mix together the granulated sugar and ground cinnamon.

4. Sprinkle the cinnamon-sugar mixture evenly over both sides of the tortillas.

5. Stack the tortillas on top of each other and cut them into wedges using a pizza cutter or knife.

6. Arrange the tortilla wedges in a single layer on the prepared baking sheet.

7. Bake in the preheated oven for 8-10 minutes, or until the chips are golden brown and crispy.

8. Remove from the oven and let cool slightly before serving.

9. Serve your Cinnamon Tortilla Chips with fruit salsa, yogurt dip, or enjoy them on their own.

10. Enjoy!

Nutritional Values (Approximate, per serving):

- Calories: 120-150 kcal

- Protein: 2-3 grams

- Fat: 5-7 grams

- Carbohydrates: 15-20 grams

- Dietary Fiber: 1-2 grams

- Sugars: 3-4 grams

Sweet and Spicy Kettle Corn:

Prep Time: 5 minutes

Cook Time: 5 minutes

Servings: 4

Ingredients:

- 1/4 cup popcorn kernels

- 2 tablespoons vegetable oil

- 2 tablespoons granulated sugar

- 1/2 teaspoon salt

- 1/4 teaspoon cayenne pepper (optional)

Instructions:

1. Heat the vegetable oil in a large pot over medium heat.

2. Add the popcorn kernels to the pot and cover with a lid.

3. Shake the pot occasionally to prevent the kernels from burning.

4. Once the popping slows down, remove the pot from the heat and let it sit for a minute to allow any remaining kernels to pop.

5. In a small bowl, mix together the granulated sugar, salt, and cayenne pepper (if using).

6. Drizzle the sugar mixture over the popped popcorn and toss to coat evenly.

7. Spread the Sweet and Spicy Kettle Corn out on a baking sheet to cool.

8. Once cooled, transfer to a serving bowl and enjoy as a delicious snack.

9. Store any leftovers in an airtight container for up to 2 days.

10. Enjoy!

Nutritional Values (Approximate, per serving):

- Calories: 120-150 kcal

- Protein: 2-3 grams

- Fat: 5-7 grams

- Carbohydrates: 15-20 grams

- Dietary Fiber: 2-3 grams

- Sugars: 6-8 grams

Blueberries and Cream Ice Pops:

Prep Time: 10 minutes

Freeze Time: 4-6 hours

Servings: 6

Ingredients:

- 1 cup fresh blueberries

- 1 cup plain Greek yogurt

- 1/4 cup honey or maple syrup

- 1 teaspoon vanilla extract

Instructions:

1. In a blender, combine the fresh blueberries, Greek yogurt, honey or maple syrup, and vanilla extract.

2. Blend until smooth and well combined.

3. Pour the mixture into ice pop molds, leaving a little space at the top for expansion.

4. Insert ice pop sticks into each mold.

5. Place the molds in the freezer and freeze for 4-6 hours, or until the ice pops are completely frozen.

6. Once frozen, remove the molds from the freezer and run them under warm water for a few seconds to loosen the ice pops.

7. Gently remove the ice pops from the molds and serve immediately.

8. Enjoy these refreshing Blueberries and Cream Ice Pops on a hot day!

Nutritional Values (Approximate, per serving):

- Calories: 70-90 kcal

- Protein: 3-4 grams

- Fat: 1-2 grams

- Carbohydrates: 12-15 grams

- Dietary Fiber: 1-2 grams

- Sugars: 9-11 grams

Candied Ginger Ice Milk:

Prep Time: 5 minutes

Freeze Time: 4-6 hours

Servings: 4

Ingredients:

- 2 cups milk (any type you prefer)

- 1/4 cup honey or maple syrup

- 1/4 cup candied ginger, finely chopped

Instructions:

1. In a blender, combine the milk, honey or maple syrup, and candied ginger.

2. Blend until the ingredients are well mixed.

3. Pour the mixture into a shallow dish or ice cube tray.

4. Place the dish or tray in the freezer and freeze for 4-6 hours, or until the mixture is semi-frozen.

5. Remove the dish or tray from the freezer and break the semi-frozen mixture into chunks.

6. Transfer the chunks to a blender and blend until smooth and creamy.

7. Pour the blended mixture back into the dish or tray and return it to the freezer.

8. Freeze for an additional 2-3 hours, or until the ice milk is completely frozen.

9. Once frozen, scoop the Candied Ginger Ice Milk into bowls and serve immediately.

10. Enjoy this unique and refreshing frozen treat!

Nutritional Values (Approximate, per serving):

- Calories: 130-150 kcal

- Protein: 4-5 grams

- Fat: 2-3 grams

- Carbohydrates: 22-25 grams

- Dietary Fiber: 0 grams

- Sugars: 20-22 grams

Meringue Cookies:

Prep **Time:** 15 minutes

Cook **Time:** 1 hour

Servings: 24 cookies

Ingredients:

- 3 large egg whites, at room temperature
- 3/4 cup granulated sugar
- 1/4 teaspoon cream of tartar
- 1/2 teaspoon vanilla extract
- Food coloring (optional)

Instructions:

1. Preheat the oven to 200°F (95°C). Line a baking sheet with parchment paper.
2. In a clean, dry mixing bowl, beat the egg whites on medium speed until foamy.
3. Add the cream of tartar and continue to beat until soft peaks form.
4. Gradually add the sugar, 1 tablespoon at a time, while continuing to beat on high speed until stiff, glossy peaks form.
5. Beat in the vanilla extract and food coloring (if using) until well incorporated.
6. Transfer the meringue mixture to a piping bag fitted with a star tip (or a plastic bag with a corner snipped off).
7. Pipe the meringue onto the prepared baking sheet in small swirls or dollops, leaving space between each cookie.
8. Bake in the preheated oven for 1 hour, or until the cookies are dry to the touch and lift easily off the parchment paper.
9. Turn off the oven and leave the cookies inside with the door closed for another hour to cool completely and dry out further.
10. Once cooled, store the meringue cookies in an airtight container at room temperature for up to 1 week.

Nutritional Values (Approximate, per serving):

- Calories: 20-25 kcal

- Protein: 0 grams

- Fat: 0 grams

- Carbohydrates: 5-6 grams

- Dietary Fiber: 0 grams

- Sugars: 5-6 grams

Corn Bread:

Prep Time: 10 minutes

Cook Time: 20-25 minutes

Servings: 12 slices

Ingredients:

- 1 cup yellow cornmeal

- 1 cup all-purpose flour

- 1/4 cup granulated sugar

- 1 tablespoon baking powder

- 1/2 teaspoon salt

- 1 cup milk

- 2 large eggs

- 1/4 cup unsalted butter, melted

Instructions:

1. Preheat the oven to 400°F (200°C). Grease a 9x9-inch baking dish or line it with parchment paper.

2. In a large mixing bowl, whisk together the cornmeal, flour, sugar, baking powder, and salt until well combined.

3. In a separate bowl, whisk together the milk, eggs, and melted butter.

4. Pour the wet ingredients into the dry ingredients and stir until just combined. Do not overmix; a few lumps are okay.

5. Pour the batter into the prepared baking dish and spread it out evenly.

6. Bake in the preheated oven for 20-25 minutes, or until the cornbread is golden brown and a toothpick inserted into the center comes out clean.

7. Remove from the oven and let cool in the baking dish for 5-10 minutes before slicing and serving.

8. Serve warm as a side dish or snack.

Nutritional Values (Approximate, per serving):

- Calories: 150-180 kcal

- Protein: 4-5 grams

- Fat: 5-6 grams

- Carbohydrates: 25-30 grams

- Dietary Fiber: 1-2 grams

- Sugars: 6-8 grams

Prep Time: 15 minutes

Cook Time: 15 minutes

Servings: 6 crostini

Ingredients:

- 1 red bell pepper
- 1 cooked chicken breast, shredded
- 6 slices of baguette or Italian bread
- 2 tablespoons olive oil
- 1 clove garlic, minced
- Salt and pepper, to taste
- Fresh basil leaves, for garnish (optional)

Instructions:

1. Preheat the oven to 400°F (200°C).
2. Place the red bell pepper on a baking sheet and roast in the oven for 15-20 minutes, or until the skin is charred and blistered.
3. Remove the pepper from the oven and place it in a bowl. Cover the bowl with plastic wrap and let it steam for 10 minutes.
4. Peel the skin off the pepper, remove the seeds, and slice it into thin strips.
5. In a small bowl, mix the shredded chicken with minced garlic, salt, and pepper.
6. Brush the slices of baguette with olive oil and toast them in the oven until golden brown.
7. Top each toasted baguette slice with shredded chicken and roasted red pepper strips.
8. Garnish with fresh basil leaves, if desired, and serve immediately.

Nutritional Values (Approximate, per serving):

- Calories: 150-180 kcal
- Protein: 10-12 grams
- Fat: 6-8 grams

- Carbohydrates: 15-18 grams

- Dietary Fiber: 1-2 grams

- Sugars: 1-2 grams

Cucumber-Wrapped Vegetable Rolls:

Prep Time: 20 minutes

Cook Time: 0 minutes

Servings: 6 rolls

Ingredients:

- 1 large cucumber

- 1/2 cup hummus

- 1/2 cup shredded carrots

- 1/2 cup sliced bell pepper (red, yellow, or orange)

- 1/2 cup sliced cucumber

- 1/4 cup sliced red onion

- Fresh parsley or cilantro, for garnish (optional)

Instructions:

1. Using a vegetable peeler or mandoline slicer, slice the cucumber lengthwise into thin strips.

2. Spread a thin layer of hummus onto each cucumber strip.

3. Place a small amount of shredded carrots, sliced bell pepper, cucumber, and red onion on one end of each cucumber strip.

4. Roll up the cucumber strip tightly around the vegetables to form a roll.

5. Secure the roll with a toothpick if necessary.

6. Repeat the process with the remaining cucumber strips and vegetables.

7. Garnish with fresh parsley or cilantro, if desired, and serve chilled.

Nutritional Values (Approximate, per serving):

- Calories: 40-50 kcal

- Protein: 1-2 grams

- Fat: 2-3 grams

- Carbohydrates: 5-6 grams

- Dietary Fiber: 1-2 grams

- Sugars: 2-3 grams

Antojitos:

| Prep | Time: | 15 | minutes |
| Cook | Time: | 10 | minutes |

Servings: 4

Ingredients:

- 8 small corn tortillas

- 1 cup refried beans

- 1 cup shredded cooked chicken

- 1 cup shredded lettuce

- 1/2 cup diced tomatoes

- 1/2 cup shredded cheese

- 1/4 cup chopped cilantro

- 1 avocado, sliced

- Lime wedges, for serving

- Salsa, for serving

Instructions:

1. Preheat a skillet over medium heat.

2. Warm the corn tortillas in the skillet for about 1 minute on each side, or until they are heated through and slightly crispy.

3. Spread a layer of refried beans onto each tortilla.

4. Top with shredded chicken, lettuce, diced tomatoes, shredded cheese, chopped cilantro, and avocado slices.

5. Squeeze fresh lime juice over the top and serve with salsa on the side.

6. Roll up the tortillas and serve immediately.

Nutritional Values (Approximate, per serving):

- Calories: 300-350 kcal

- Protein: 15-18 grams

- Fat: 12-15 grams

- Carbohydrates: 30-35 grams

- Dietary Fiber: 6-8 grams

- Sugars: 2-3 grams

Prep **Time**: 20 minutes

Cook **Time**: 10 minutes

Servings: 4

Ingredients:

- 2 boneless, skinless chicken breasts, cut into cubes
- 1 red bell pepper, cut into chunks
- 1 yellow bell pepper, cut into chunks
- 1 red onion, cut into chunks
- 1 zucchini, sliced
- 1/4 cup olive oil
- 2 tablespoons balsamic vinegar
- 2 cloves garlic, minced
- 1 teaspoon dried oregano
- Salt and pepper, to taste
- Wooden skewers, soaked in water for 30 minutes

Instructions:

1. In a small bowl, whisk together olive oil, balsamic vinegar, minced garlic, dried oregano, salt, and pepper to make the marinade.

2. Place the chicken cubes in a shallow dish and pour the marinade over them. Toss to coat the chicken evenly. Cover and refrigerate for at least 1 hour.

3. Preheat the grill to medium-high heat.

4. Thread the marinated chicken cubes, bell pepper chunks, onion chunks, and zucchini slices onto the soaked wooden skewers, alternating between ingredients.

5. Grill the kebabs for 8-10 minutes, turning occasionally, or until the chicken is cooked through and the vegetables are tender.

6. Remove from the grill and serve immediately.

Nutritional Values (Approximate, per serving):

- Calories: 250-300 kcal
- Protein: 20-25 grams
- Fat: 10-12 grams
- Carbohydrates: 15-18 grams
- Dietary Fiber: 3-5 grams
- Sugars: 5-7 grams

<h1 style="text-align:center">Five-Spice Chicken Lettuce Wraps:</h1>

Prep Time: 15 minutes

Cook Time: 10 minutes

Servings: 4

Ingredients:

- 1 lb ground chicken
- 1 tablespoon vegetable oil
- 2 cloves garlic, minced
- 1 small onion, finely chopped
- 1 teaspoon five-spice powder
- 1 tablespoon soy sauce
- 1 tablespoon hoisin sauce
- 1 teaspoon sesame oil
- 1 teaspoon rice vinegar
- 1 teaspoon Sriracha sauce (optional)
- Salt and pepper, to taste
- 1 head iceberg lettuce, leaves separated
- 1/4 cup chopped green onions
- 1/4 cup chopped fresh cilantro
- 1/4 cup chopped peanuts (optional)

Instructions:

1. Heat vegetable oil in a large skillet over medium heat. Add minced garlic and chopped onion, and sauté until softened, about 2-3 minutes.

2. Add ground chicken to the skillet, breaking it apart with a spatula. Cook until browned and no longer pink, about 5-6 minutes.

3. Stir in five-spice powder, soy sauce, hoisin sauce, sesame oil, rice vinegar, and Sriracha sauce (if using). Season with salt and pepper to taste. Cook for an additional 2-3 minutes, stirring occasionally.

4. Remove the skillet from heat and let the chicken mixture cool slightly.

5. To serve, spoon the chicken mixture onto individual lettuce leaves. Top with chopped green onions, fresh cilantro, and chopped peanuts (if using).

6. Roll up the lettuce leaves and enjoy these flavorful Five-Spice Chicken Lettuce Wraps!

Nutritional Values (Approximate, per serving):

- Calories: 250-300 kcal

- Protein: 20-25 grams

- Fat: 10-12 grams

- Carbohydrates: 10-12 grams

- Dietary Fiber: 2-3 grams

- Sugars: 4-6 grams

CHAPTER EIGHT:

Satisfying Entrees with Flavorful Twists

Grilled Shrimp with Cucumber Lime Salsa:

Prep Time: 15 minutes

Cook Time: 5 minutes

Servings: 4

Ingredients:

- 1 lb large shrimp, peeled and deveined
- 2 tablespoons olive oil
- Salt and pepper, to taste
- 1 cucumber, diced
- 1 tomato, diced
- 1/4 red onion, finely chopped
- 1 jalapeño pepper, seeded and minced
- 2 tablespoons fresh cilantro, chopped
- Juice of 2 limes
- 1 tablespoon honey or agave syrup
- 1 tablespoon olive oil

Instructions:

1. Preheat the grill to medium-high heat.
2. In a bowl, toss the shrimp with olive oil, salt, and pepper until evenly coated.
3. Thread the shrimp onto skewers, then grill for 2-3 minutes per side until cooked through and slightly charred.
4. While the shrimp are grilling, prepare the cucumber lime salsa. In a separate bowl, combine diced cucumber, tomato, red onion, jalapeño pepper, and cilantro.

5. In a small jar or bowl, whisk together lime juice, honey or agave syrup, and olive oil to make the dressing. Pour the dressing over the cucumber salsa and toss to coat.

6. Once the shrimp are cooked, remove them from the grill and transfer to a serving platter.

7. Serve the grilled shrimp with the cucumber lime salsa on the side.

8. Enjoy this light and refreshing dish!

Nutritional Values (Approximate, per serving):

- Calories: 200-250 kcal
- Protein: 20-25 grams
- Fat: 10-12 grams
- Carbohydrates: 8-10 grams
- Dietary Fiber: 2-3 grams
- Sugars: 4-6 grams

Prep **Time:** 15 minutes

Cook **Time:** 15 minutes

Servings: 4

Ingredients:

- 8 oz linguine pasta
- 1 lb large shrimp, peeled and deveined
- 4 cloves garlic, minced
- 1/4 cup unsalted butter
- 1/4 cup white wine
- 2 tablespoons lemon juice
- Zest of 1 lemon
- 1/4 cup chopped fresh parsley
- Salt and pepper, to taste
- Red pepper flakes, to taste (optional)
- Grated Parmesan cheese, for serving

Instructions:

1. Cook the linguine pasta according to package Instructions until al dente. Drain and set aside.

2. In a large skillet, melt the butter over medium heat. Add the minced garlic and cook for 1-2 minutes until fragrant.

3. Add the shrimp to the skillet and cook for 2-3 minutes on each side until pink and cooked through.

4. Stir in the white wine, lemon juice, lemon zest, and chopped parsley. Season with salt, pepper, and red pepper flakes if desired.

5. Add the cooked linguine to the skillet and toss to coat the pasta in the shrimp scampi sauce.

6. Serve the shrimp scampi linguine immediately, garnished with grated Parmesan cheese.

7. Enjoy this delicious and flavorful dish!

Nutritional Values (Approximate, per serving):

- Calories: 350-400 kcal

- Protein: 20-25 grams

- Fat: 15-18 grams

- Carbohydrates: 30-35 grams

- Dietary Fiber: 2-3 grams

- Sugars: 1-2 grams

Crab Cakes with Lime Salsa:

| **Prep** | **Time:** | 20 | minutes |
| **Cook** | **Time:** | 10 | minutes |

Servings: 4

Ingredients: For the crab cakes:

- 1 lb lump crab meat

- 1/2 cup breadcrumbs

- 1/4 cup mayonnaise

- 1 egg

- 2 tablespoons chopped fresh parsley

- 1 tablespoon Dijon mustard

- 1 teaspoon Old Bay seasoning

- Salt and pepper, to taste

- 2 tablespoons olive oil

For the lime salsa:

- 2 tomatoes, diced

- 1/2 red onion, finely chopped

- 1 jalapeño pepper, seeded and minced

- Juice of 2 limes

- Zest of 1 lime

- 2 tablespoons chopped fresh cilantro

- Salt and pepper, to taste

Instructions:

1. In a large bowl, combine lump crab meat, breadcrumbs, mayonnaise, egg, chopped parsley, Dijon mustard, Old Bay seasoning, salt, and pepper. Mix until well combined.

2. Divide the crab mixture into equal portions and shape into crab cakes.

3. Heat olive oil in a skillet over medium heat. Cook the crab cakes for 3-4 minutes on each side until golden brown and heated through.

4. While the crab cakes are cooking, prepare the lime salsa. In a bowl, combine diced tomatoes, finely chopped red onion, minced jalapeño pepper, lime juice, lime zest, chopped cilantro, salt, and pepper.

5. Serve the crab cakes with the lime salsa on top or on the side.

6. Enjoy these flavorful crab cakes with a zesty lime salsa!

Nutritional Values (Approximate, per serving):

- Calories: 300-350 kcal (crab cakes only)

- Protein: 20-25 grams

- Fat: 15-18 grams

- Carbohydrates: 15-20 grams

- Dietary Fiber: 2-3 grams

- Sugars: 2-3 grams

Prep **Time:** 20 minutes

Cook **Time:** 30 minutes

Servings: 6

Ingredients:

- 1 lb mixed seafood (shrimp, scallops, crab meat, etc.), thawed if frozen
- 2 cups cooked rice
- 1 onion, diced
- 2 cloves garlic, minced
- 1 red bell pepper, diced
- 1 green bell pepper, diced
- 1 cup frozen peas
- 1 cup sliced mushrooms
- 1 cup seafood or chicken broth
- 1 cup heavy cream
- 1/4 cup all-purpose flour
- 2 tablespoons butter
- 2 tablespoons olive oil
- Salt and pepper, to taste
- 1/2 cup grated Parmesan cheese
- Chopped fresh parsley, for garnish

Instructions:

1. Preheat the oven to 375°F (190°C). Grease a casserole dish with butter or cooking spray.

2. In a large skillet, heat olive oil over medium heat. Add diced onion and minced garlic, and sauté until softened.

3. Add diced bell peppers, frozen peas, and sliced mushrooms to the skillet. Cook for 5-7 minutes until vegetables are tender.

4. In a separate saucepan, melt butter over medium heat. Stir in all-purpose flour to create a roux. Cook for 1-2 minutes until lightly golden.

5. Gradually whisk in seafood or chicken broth and heavy cream until smooth. Cook until the sauce thickens, stirring constantly.

6. Season the sauce with salt and pepper to taste. Remove from heat and set aside.

7. In the prepared casserole dish, layer cooked rice, mixed seafood, and sautéed vegetables.

8. Pour the prepared sauce over the seafood and vegetables in the casserole dish.

9. Sprinkle grated Parmesan cheese evenly over the top.

10. Cover the casserole dish with aluminum foil and bake in the preheated oven for 20-25 minutes.

11. Remove the foil and bake for an additional 5-10 minutes until the casserole is bubbly and golden brown on top.

12. Garnish with chopped fresh parsley before serving.

13. Enjoy this delicious seafood casserole as a comforting and satisfying meal!

Nutritional Values (Approximate, per serving):

- Calories: 400-450 kcal

- Protein: 25-30 grams

- Fat: 20-25 grams

- Carbohydrates: 30-35 grams

- Dietary Fiber: 3-5 grams

- Sugars: 3-5 grams

| **Prep** | **Time:** | 10 | minutes |
| **Cook** | **Time:** | 15 | minutes |

Servings: 4

Ingredients:

- 4 salmon fillets
- 1/4 cup honey
- 2 tablespoons soy sauce
- 1 tablespoon olive oil
- 2 cloves garlic, minced
- 1 teaspoon grated ginger
- 1 teaspoon sesame oil
- Salt and pepper, to taste
- Sesame seeds, for garnish
- Chopped green onions, for garnish

Instructions:

1. Preheat the oven to 400°F (200°C). Line a baking sheet with parchment paper or foil.
2. In a small bowl, whisk together honey, soy sauce, olive oil, minced garlic, grated ginger, sesame oil, salt, and pepper to make the glaze.
3. Place the salmon fillets on the prepared baking sheet.
4. Brush the glaze generously over the salmon fillets, coating them evenly.
5. Bake the salmon in the preheated oven for 12-15 minutes, or until the fish flakes easily with a fork.
6. Remove the salmon from the oven and transfer to a serving platter.
7. Garnish with sesame seeds and chopped green onions.
8. Serve the sweet glazed salmon hot with your favorite side dishes.
9. Enjoy this flavorful and nutritious dish!

Nutritional Values (Approximate, per serving):

- Calories: 300-350 kcal

- Protein: 25-30 grams

- Fat: 15-18 grams

- Carbohydrates: 10-12 grams

- Dietary Fiber: 0-1 grams

- Sugars: 10-12 grams

Herb-Crusted Baked Haddock:

Prep Time: 10 minutes

Cook Time: 20 minutes

Servings: 4

Ingredients:

- 4 haddock fillets

- 1/2 cup breadcrumbs

- 2 tablespoons grated Parmesan cheese

- 1 tablespoon chopped fresh parsley

- 1 teaspoon dried oregano

- 1 teaspoon dried thyme

- 1 teaspoon dried basil

- 1/2 teaspoon garlic powder

- 1/4 teaspoon paprika

- Salt and pepper, to taste

- 2 tablespoons melted butter or olive oil

- Lemon wedges, for serving

Instructions:

1. Preheat the oven to 400°F (200°C). Line a baking sheet with parchment paper or foil.

2. In a shallow dish, combine breadcrumbs, grated Parmesan cheese, chopped fresh parsley, dried oregano, dried thyme, dried basil, garlic powder, paprika, salt, and pepper.

3. Pat the haddock fillets dry with paper towels. Dip each fillet into the melted butter or olive oil, then coat evenly with the herb and breadcrumb mixture, pressing gently to adhere.

4. Place the coated haddock fillets on the prepared baking sheet.

5. Bake in the preheated oven for 15-20 minutes, or until the fish is opaque and flakes easily with a fork.

6. Remove from the oven and serve immediately with lemon wedges.

7. Enjoy this delicious herb-crusted baked haddock as a flavorful and healthy seafood dish!

Nutritional Values (Approximate, per serving):

- Calories: 200-250 kcal

- Protein: 20-25 grams

- Fat: 10-12 grams

- Carbohydrates: 5-7 grams

- Dietary Fiber: 1-2 grams

- Sugars: 0-1 grams

Prep **Time:** 10 minutes

Cook **Time:** 10 minutes

Servings: 4

Ingredients:

- 4 sole fillets
- 1/2 cup all-purpose flour
- 2 eggs, beaten
- 1 cup breadcrumbs
- 1 teaspoon dried dill
- 1 teaspoon dried parsley
- 1/2 teaspoon garlic powder
- 1/2 teaspoon onion powder
- Salt and pepper, to taste
- 2 tablespoons olive oil or melted butter
- Lemon wedges, for serving

Instructions:

1. Place the all-purpose flour, beaten eggs, and breadcrumbs in separate shallow dishes.
2. Season the breadcrumbs with dried dill, dried parsley, garlic powder, onion powder, salt, and pepper, and mix well.
3. Pat the sole fillets dry with paper towels. Dredge each fillet in the flour, shaking off any excess.
4. Dip the floured fillets into the beaten eggs, then coat evenly with the seasoned breadcrumbs, pressing gently to adhere.
5. Heat olive oil or melted butter in a large skillet over medium heat.
6. Add the breaded sole fillets to the skillet and cook for 3-4 minutes on each side, or until golden brown and cooked through.
7. Remove from the skillet and drain on paper towels to remove excess oil.

8. Serve the shore lunch–style sole hot with lemon wedges on the side.

9. Enjoy this classic and comforting fish dish reminiscent of a traditional shore lunch!

Nutritional Values (Approximate, per serving):

- Calories: 250-300 kcal

- Protein: 20-25 grams

- Fat: 10-12 grams

- Carbohydrates: 15-20 grams

- Dietary Fiber: 1-2 grams

- Sugars: 1-2 grams

| Prep | Time: | 10 | minutes |
| Cook | Time: | 15 | minutes |

Servings: 4

Ingredients:

- 4 cod fillets
- 1 tablespoon olive oil
- Salt and pepper, to taste
- 1 cucumber, diced
- 2 tablespoons chopped fresh dill
- 1 tablespoon finely chopped red onion
- 1 tablespoon lemon juice
- 1 tablespoon extra virgin olive oil
- Salt and pepper, to taste

Instructions:

1. Preheat the oven to 400°F (200°C). Line a baking sheet with parchment paper.
2. Place the cod fillets on the prepared baking sheet. Drizzle olive oil over the fillets and season with salt and pepper.
3. Bake in the preheated oven for 12-15 minutes, or until the cod is cooked through and flakes easily with a fork.
4. While the cod is baking, prepare the cucumber-dill salsa. In a mixing bowl, combine diced cucumber, chopped fresh dill, finely chopped red onion, lemon juice, extra virgin olive oil, salt, and pepper. Toss to combine.
5. Once the cod is cooked, remove from the oven and transfer to serving plates.
6. Top each cod fillet with cucumber-dill salsa.
7. Serve immediately, garnished with additional fresh dill if desired.
8. Enjoy this flavorful and nutritious baked cod with cucumber-dill salsa!

Nutritional Values (Approximate, per serving):

- Calories: 200-250 kcal

- Protein: 20-25 grams

- Fat: 10-12 grams

- Carbohydrates: 5-7 grams

- Dietary Fiber: 1-2 grams

- Sugars: 2-3 grams

Cilantro-Lime Flounder:

Prep Time: 10 minutes

Cook Time: 10 minutes

Servings: 4

Ingredients:

- 4 flounder fillets

- 2 tablespoons olive oil

- Zest and juice of 1 lime

- 2 cloves garlic, minced

- 2 tablespoons chopped fresh cilantro

- Salt and pepper, to taste

- Lime wedges, for serving

Instructions:

1. Preheat the oven to 400°F (200°C). Line a baking sheet with parchment paper.

2. Place the flounder fillets on the prepared baking sheet. Drizzle olive oil over the fillets.

3. In a small bowl, combine lime zest, lime juice, minced garlic, chopped fresh cilantro, salt, and pepper. Mix well.

4. Spoon the cilantro-lime mixture over the flounder fillets, spreading it evenly.

5. Bake in the preheated oven for 8-10 minutes, or until the flounder is opaque and flakes easily with a fork.

6. Remove from the oven and transfer the flounder to serving plates.

7. Serve immediately with lime wedges on the side.

8. Enjoy this light and zesty cilantro-lime flounder as a delightful seafood dish!

Nutritional Values (Approximate, per serving):

- Calories: 150-200 kcal

- Protein: 20-25 grams

- Fat: 8-10 grams

- Carbohydrates: 2-3 grams

- Dietary Fiber: 0-1 gram

- Sugars: 0-1 gram

Herb Pesto Tuna:

Prep **Time:** 10 minutes

Cook **Time:** 10 minutes

Servings: 4

Ingredients:

- 4 tuna steaks
- Salt and pepper, to taste
- 2 tablespoons olive oil
- 1/4 cup chopped fresh basil
- 1/4 cup chopped fresh parsley
- 2 cloves garlic, minced
- 2 tablespoons pine nuts
- 1/4 cup grated Parmesan cheese
- Juice of 1 lemon

Instructions:

1. Season the tuna steaks with salt and pepper on both sides.
2. In a small bowl, combine the chopped basil, chopped parsley, minced garlic, pine nuts, grated Parmesan cheese, and lemon juice. Mix well to form a paste.
3. Heat olive oil in a skillet over medium-high heat.
4. Add the seasoned tuna steaks to the skillet and cook for 3-4 minutes on each side, or until desired doneness.
5. Remove the tuna steaks from the skillet and transfer to serving plates.
6. Spoon the herb pesto mixture over the cooked tuna steaks.
7. Serve immediately, garnished with additional chopped herbs if desired.
8. Enjoy this flavorful herb pesto tuna as a delicious seafood dish!

Nutritional Values (Approximate, per serving):

- Calories: 250-300 kcal
- Protein: 30-35 grams

- Fat: 12-15 grams

- Carbohydrates: 2-3 grams

- Dietary Fiber: 0-1 gram

- Sugars: 0 grams

Grilled Calamari with Lemon and Herbs:

Prep Time: 15 minutes

Cook Time: 5 minutes

Servings: 4

Ingredients:

- 1 lb calamari tubes, cleaned and sliced into rings

- 2 tablespoons olive oil

- 2 cloves garlic, minced

- Zest and juice of 1 lemon

- 2 tablespoons chopped fresh parsley

- Salt and pepper, to taste

- Lemon wedges, for serving

Instructions:

1. In a bowl, combine the sliced calamari rings, olive oil, minced garlic, lemon zest, lemon juice, chopped parsley, salt, and pepper. Toss to coat the calamari evenly.

2. Preheat a grill or grill pan over medium-high heat.

3. Thread the marinated calamari rings onto skewers or place them directly on the grill.

4. Grill the calamari for 1-2 minutes on each side, or until lightly charred and cooked through.

5. Remove the grilled calamari from the heat and transfer to a serving platter.

6. Serve immediately with lemon wedges on the side.

7. Enjoy this tender and flavorful grilled calamari as a delightful seafood appetizer or main dish!

Nutritional Values (Approximate, per serving):

- Calories: 150-200 kcal
- Protein: 20-25 grams
- Fat: 8-10 grams
- Carbohydrates: 2-3 grams
- Dietary Fiber: 0 grams
- Sugars: 0 grams

Lemon-Herb Chicken:

Prep **Time:** 10 minutes

Cook **Time:** 20 minutes

Servings: 4

Ingredients:

- 4 boneless, skinless chicken breasts
- 2 tablespoons olive oil
- 2 cloves garlic, minced
- Zest and juice of 1 lemon
- 1 tablespoon chopped fresh thyme
- 1 tablespoon chopped fresh rosemary
- Salt and pepper, to taste

Instructions:

1. Preheat the oven to 375°F (190°C).
2. In a small bowl, whisk together the olive oil, minced garlic, lemon zest, lemon juice, chopped thyme, and chopped rosemary.
3. Season the chicken breasts with salt and pepper on both sides.
4. Place the seasoned chicken breasts in a baking dish.
5. Pour the lemon-herb mixture over the chicken breasts, ensuring they are evenly coated.
6. Bake in the preheated oven for 20-25 minutes, or until the chicken is cooked through and no longer pink in the center.
7. Remove the chicken from the oven and let it rest for a few minutes before serving.
8. Serve the lemon-herb chicken hot with your favorite side dishes.
9. Enjoy this flavorful and aromatic chicken dish!

Nutritional Values (Approximate, per serving):

- Calories: 250-300 kcal

- Protein: 30-35 grams

- Fat: 10-12 grams

- Carbohydrates: 2-3 grams

- Dietary Fiber: 0 grams

- Sugars: 0 grams

Asian Chicken Satay:

Prep Time: 15 minutes

Cook Time: 10 minutes

Servings: 4

Ingredients:

- 1 lb boneless, skinless chicken breasts, cut into thin strips

- 1/4 cup soy sauce

- 2 tablespoons honey

- 2 cloves garlic, minced

- 1 tablespoon grated ginger

- 2 tablespoons lime juice

- 1 tablespoon sesame oil

- 1 teaspoon chili flakes (optional)

- Bamboo skewers, soaked in water for 30 minutes

- Chopped peanuts and chopped cilantro, for garnish (optional)

Instructions:

1. In a bowl, whisk together the soy sauce, honey, minced garlic, grated ginger, lime juice, sesame oil, and chili flakes (if using) to make the marinade.

2. Add the chicken strips to the marinade and toss to coat. Cover the bowl and refrigerate for at least 30 minutes, or up to 2 hours.

3. Preheat the grill or grill pan over medium-high heat.

4. Thread the marinated chicken strips onto the soaked bamboo skewers.

5. Grill the chicken skewers for 4-5 minutes on each side, or until cooked through and lightly charred.

6. Remove the chicken skewers from the grill and transfer to a serving platter.

7. Garnish with chopped peanuts and chopped cilantro, if desired.

8. Serve the Asian chicken satay hot with peanut sauce or your favorite dipping sauce.

9. Enjoy these flavorful and tender chicken skewers as an appetizer or main dish!

Nutritional Values (Approximate, per serving):

- Calories: 200-250 kcal

- Protein: 25-30 grams

- Fat: 8-10 grams

- Carbohydrates: 8-10 grams

- Dietary Fiber: 0-1 gram

- Sugars: 6-8 grams

Chicken Stir-Fry:

| **Prep** | **Time:** | 15 | minutes |
| **Cook** | **Time:** | 10 | minutes |

Servings: 4

Ingredients:

- 1 lb boneless, skinless chicken breasts, thinly sliced

- 2 tablespoons soy sauce

- 1 tablespoon oyster sauce

- 1 tablespoon hoisin sauce

- 1 tablespoon sesame oil

- 2 tablespoons vegetable oil

- 2 cloves garlic, minced

- 1 tablespoon grated ginger

- 1 onion, thinly sliced

- 1 bell pepper, thinly sliced

- 1 cup broccoli florets

- 1 carrot, thinly sliced

- Salt and pepper, to taste

- Cooked rice or noodles, for serving

- Chopped green onions and sesame seeds, for garnish (optional)

Instructions:

1. In a bowl, combine the sliced chicken breasts with soy sauce, oyster sauce, and hoisin sauce. Toss to coat the chicken evenly and set aside to marinate for 10-15 minutes.

2. Heat sesame oil and vegetable oil in a large skillet or wok over medium-high heat.

3. Add minced garlic and grated ginger to the hot oil and stir-fry for about 30 seconds until fragrant.

4. Add the marinated chicken to the skillet and stir-fry for 3-4 minutes until cooked through and lightly browned.

5. Push the chicken to one side of the skillet and add sliced onion, bell pepper, broccoli florets, and sliced carrot. Stir-fry the vegetables for 2-3 minutes until slightly softened.

6. Season the stir-fry with salt and pepper to taste, and toss everything together.

7. Remove the skillet from heat and transfer the chicken stir-fry to a serving platter.

8. Serve the chicken stir-fry hot with cooked rice or noodles.

9. Garnish with chopped green onions and sesame seeds, if desired.

10. Enjoy this delicious and colorful chicken stir-fry as a quick and easy meal!

Nutritional Values (Approximate, per serving):

- Calories: 250-300 kcal

- Protein: 25-30 grams

- Fat: 10-12 grams

- Carbohydrates: 15-20 grams

- Dietary Fiber: 3-4 grams

- Sugars: 5-7 grams

Indian Chicken Curry:

Prep   **Time:**   15   minutes

Cook   **Time:**   25   minutes

Servings: 4

Ingredients:

- 1 lb boneless, skinless chicken thighs, cut into bite-sized pieces
- 2 tablespoons vegetable oil
- 1 onion, finely chopped
- 2 cloves garlic, minced
- 1 tablespoon grated ginger
- 2 tomatoes, finely chopped
- 2 tablespoons tomato paste
- 1 teaspoon ground cumin
- 1 teaspoon ground coriander
- 1/2 teaspoon ground turmeric
- 1/2 teaspoon paprika
- 1/4 teaspoon cayenne pepper (adjust to taste)
- 1 cup coconut milk
- Salt and pepper, to taste
- Chopped fresh cilantro, for garnish
- Cooked rice or naan, for serving

Instructions:

1. Heat vegetable oil in a large skillet or pot over medium heat.
2. Add chopped onion to the hot oil and sauté for 2-3 minutes until softened.
3. Stir in minced garlic and grated ginger, and cook for another minute until fragrant.

4. Add the chopped tomatoes and tomato paste to the skillet, and cook for 5-6 minutes until the tomatoes break down and form a thick sauce.

5. Stir in ground cumin, ground coriander, ground turmeric, paprika, and cayenne pepper. Cook for 1-2 minutes until the spices are fragrant.

6. Add the bite-sized chicken pieces to the skillet and stir to coat them with the spice mixture.

7. Pour in the coconut milk and season with salt and pepper to taste. Stir to combine.

8. Bring the curry to a simmer, then reduce the heat to low and cover the skillet. Let it cook for 15-20 minutes, stirring occasionally, until the chicken is cooked through and the flavors are well blended.

9. Remove the skillet from heat and garnish the chicken curry with chopped fresh cilantro.

10. Serve the Indian chicken curry hot with cooked rice or naan bread.

11. Enjoy this aromatic and flavorful curry as a comforting meal!

Nutritional Values (Approximate, per serving):

- Calories: 300-350 kcal
- Protein: 20-25 grams
- Fat: 15-18 grams
- Carbohydrates: 10-12 grams
- Dietary Fiber: 2-3 grams
- Sugars: 4-6 grams

Prep   **Time:**   15   minutes

Cook   **Time:**   25   minutes

Servings: 4

Ingredients:

- 4 boneless, skinless chicken breasts
- 1 onion, finely chopped
- 2 cloves garlic, minced
- 1 tablespoon olive oil
- 1 teaspoon ground turmeric
- 1 teaspoon ground cumin
- 1 teaspoon ground cinnamon
- 1/2 teaspoon ground paprika
- 1/4 teaspoon ground cloves
- Salt and pepper, to taste
- 1 cup chicken broth
- 1/4 cup lemon juice
- 1/4 cup chopped fresh cilantro or parsley, for garnish
- Cooked rice or couscous, for serving

Instructions:

1. Season the chicken breasts with salt and pepper on both sides.

2. Heat olive oil in a large skillet over medium heat. Add the chopped onion and minced garlic, and sauté until softened and fragrant, about 2-3 minutes.

3. Add the seasoned chicken breasts to the skillet and cook for 4-5 minutes on each side until golden brown.

4. In a small bowl, mix together ground turmeric, ground cumin, ground cinnamon, ground paprika, and ground cloves.

5. Sprinkle the spice mixture over the chicken breasts in the skillet, coating them evenly.

6. Pour chicken broth and lemon juice into the skillet, stirring gently to combine.

7. Reduce the heat to low, cover the skillet, and let the chicken simmer in the sauce for 15-20 minutes until cooked through and tender.

8. Once the chicken is cooked, transfer it to a serving platter.

9. Spoon some of the sauce over the chicken and garnish with chopped fresh cilantro or parsley.

10. Serve the Persian chicken hot with cooked rice or couscous.

11. Enjoy this flavorful and aromatic dish inspired by Persian cuisine!

Nutritional Values (Approximate, per serving):

- Calories: 250-300 kcal

- Protein: 25-30 grams

- Fat: 8-10 grams

- Carbohydrates: 10-12 grams

- Dietary Fiber: 2-3 grams

- Sugars: 2-3 grams

Prep **Time:** 10 minutes

Cook **Time:** 15 minutes

Servings: 4

Ingredients:

- 4 boneless pork chops
- Salt and pepper, to taste
- 1/4 cup prepared basil pesto
- 1 tablespoon olive oil
- 2 cloves garlic, minced
- 1/4 cup chicken broth or white wine
- 2 tablespoons grated Parmesan cheese, for garnish (optional)
- Fresh basil leaves, for garnish (optional)

Instructions:

1. Season the pork chops with salt and pepper on both sides.
2. Spread a thin layer of basil pesto over each pork chop, covering them evenly.
3. Heat olive oil in a large skillet over medium-high heat. Add minced garlic and sauté for about 1 minute until fragrant.
4. Place the seasoned and pesto-coated pork chops in the skillet and cook for 4-5 minutes on each side until golden brown and cooked through.
5. Pour chicken broth or white wine into the skillet, scraping up any browned bits from the bottom of the pan to deglaze.
6. Let the pork chops simmer in the sauce for another 2-3 minutes until the sauce thickens slightly.
7. Remove the skillet from heat and transfer the pork chops to a serving platter.
8. Garnish with grated Parmesan cheese and fresh basil leaves, if desired.
9. Serve the pesto pork chops hot with your favorite side dishes.
10. Enjoy these delicious and flavorful pork chops with a hint of basil pesto!

Nutritional Values (Approximate, per serving):

- Calories: 300-350 kcal

- Protein: 30-35 grams

- Fat: 15-18 grams

- Carbohydrates: 2-4 grams

- Dietary Fiber: 0 grams

- Sugars: 0 grams

Pork Souvlaki:

Prep	**Time:**	15	minutes
Marinating	**Time:**	1-2	hours
Cook	**Time:**	10	minutes

Servings: 4

Ingredients:

- 1 lb pork tenderloin, cut into 1-inch cubes

- 2 tablespoons olive oil

- 2 cloves garlic, minced

- 1 teaspoon dried oregano

- 1 teaspoon dried thyme

- 1 teaspoon dried rosemary

- Salt and pepper, to taste

- Juice of 1 lemon

- 4 pita bread rounds

- Tzatziki sauce, for serving

- Chopped fresh parsley, for garnish

Instructions:

1. In a large bowl, combine olive oil, minced garlic, dried oregano, dried thyme, dried rosemary, salt, pepper, and lemon juice.

2. Add the pork cubes to the marinade and toss until well coated. Cover and refrigerate for 1-2 hours to marinate.

3. Preheat grill or grill pan over medium-high heat.

4. Thread the marinated pork cubes onto skewers.

5. Grill the pork skewers for 3-4 minutes on each side, or until cooked through and slightly charred.

6. Warm the pita bread rounds on the grill for 1-2 minutes on each side.

7. Serve the grilled pork souvlaki on warm pita bread rounds, topped with tzatziki sauce and chopped fresh parsley.

8. Enjoy these delicious Greek-inspired pork souvlaki as a flavorful and satisfying meal!

Nutritional Values (Approximate, per serving):

- Calories: 300-350 kcal
- Protein: 25-30 grams
- Fat: 10-12 grams
- Carbohydrates: 25-30 grams
- Dietary Fiber: 2-3 grams
- Sugars: 1-2 grams

Prep	**Time:**	15	minutes
Marinating	**Time:**	2-4	hours
Cook	**Time:**	1 hour 30	minutes

Servings: 6-8

Ingredients:

- 4 lbs pork leg, bone-in
- 4 cloves garlic, minced
- 2 tablespoons olive oil
- 1 tablespoon chili powder
- 1 teaspoon smoked paprika
- 1 teaspoon cumin
- 1 teaspoon dried oregano
- 1 teaspoon salt
- 1/2 teaspoon black pepper
- Juice of 1 lime
- Lime wedges, for serving
- Chopped fresh cilantro, for garnish

Instructions:

1. In a small bowl, combine minced garlic, olive oil, chili powder, smoked paprika, cumin, dried oregano, salt, pepper, and lime juice to make the marinade.

2. Place the pork leg in a large resealable plastic bag or shallow dish. Pour the marinade over the pork leg, ensuring it is evenly coated. Marinate in the refrigerator for 2-4 hours, or overnight if possible.

3. Preheat the oven to 350°F (175°C).

4. Place the marinated pork leg on a roasting rack set in a roasting pan. Pour any remaining marinade over the pork.

5. Roast the pork leg in the preheated oven for 1 hour 30 minutes, or until the internal temperature reaches 145°F (63°C) on a meat thermometer.

6. Remove the pork leg from the oven and let it rest for 10 minutes before slicing.

7. Slice the roasted pork leg and serve with lime wedges and chopped fresh cilantro.

8. Enjoy this flavorful and tender chili-roasted pork leg as a delicious main dish!

Nutritional Values (Approximate, per serving):

- Calories: 400-450 kcal

- Protein: 35-40 grams

- Fat: 25-30 grams

- Carbohydrates: 2-4 grams

- Dietary Fiber: 0 grams

- Sugars: 0 grams

Prep Time: 15 minutes

Cook Time: 20 minutes

Servings: 4

Ingredients:

- 1 lb beef sirloin, thinly sliced
- 2 tablespoons vegetable oil
- 1 onion, thinly sliced
- 1 red bell pepper, thinly sliced
- 1 green bell pepper, thinly sliced
- 1 cup snap peas
- 2 cloves garlic, minced
- 1 tablespoon soy sauce
- 1 tablespoon oyster sauce
- 1 tablespoon hoisin sauce
- 1 teaspoon sesame oil
- Cooked rice, for serving
- Chopped green onions, for garnish

Instructions:

1. Heat vegetable oil in a large skillet over medium-high heat.

2. Add thinly sliced beef sirloin to the skillet and cook until browned, about 2-3 minutes per side. Remove beef from skillet and set aside.

3. In the same skillet, add sliced onion, red bell pepper, green bell pepper, and snap peas. Cook until vegetables are tender-crisp, about 4-5 minutes.

4. Add minced garlic to the skillet and cook for an additional 1 minute.

5. Return the cooked beef to the skillet. Stir in soy sauce, oyster sauce, hoisin sauce, and sesame oil. Cook for 2-3 minutes, stirring occasionally, until heated through.

6. Serve the beef stir-up over cooked rice, garnished with chopped green onions.

7. Enjoy this delicious open-faced beef stir-up as a flavorful and satisfying meal!

Nutritional Values (Approximate, per serving):

- Calories: 300-350 kcal
- Protein: 25-30 grams
- Fat: 15-18 grams
- Carbohydrates: 15-20 grams
- Dietary Fiber: 3-4 grams
- Sugars: 6-8 grams

Sweet and Sour Meatloaf:

Prep Time: 15 minutes

Cook Time: 1 hour

Servings: 6

Ingredients:

- 1 lb ground beef
- 1 onion, finely chopped
- 1/2 cup breadcrumbs
- 1 egg, beaten
- 1/4 cup milk
- Salt and pepper, to taste
- 1/2 cup ketchup
- 1/4 cup brown sugar
- 2 tablespoons apple cider vinegar
- 1 tablespoon Worcestershire sauce

Instructions:

1. Preheat the oven to 350°F (175°C).
2. In a large mixing bowl, combine ground beef, finely chopped onion, breadcrumbs, beaten egg, milk, salt, and pepper. Mix until well combined.
3. Shape the mixture into a loaf and place it in a greased loaf pan.
4. In a small bowl, mix together ketchup, brown sugar, apple cider vinegar, and Worcestershire sauce to make the sweet and sour glaze.
5. Spread the sweet and sour glaze evenly over the top of the meatloaf.
6. Bake the meatloaf in the preheated oven for 1 hour, or until cooked through and the internal temperature reaches 160°F (71°C).
7. Remove the meatloaf from the oven and let it rest for 5-10 minutes before slicing.
8. Serve slices of the sweet and sour meatloaf with your favorite side dishes.
9. Enjoy this classic comfort food with a sweet and tangy twist!

Nutritional Values (Approximate, per serving):

- Calories: 300-350 kcal

- Protein: 20-25 grams

- Fat: 15-20 grams

- Carbohydrates: 20-25 grams

- Dietary Fiber: 1-2 grams

- Sugars: 10-12 grams

| Prep | **Time:** | 15 | minutes |
| **Cook** | **Time**: | 10 | minutes |

Servings: 4

Ingredients:

- 4 steaks (e.g., ribeye, sirloin), about 6 oz each
- Salt and pepper, to taste
- 1 cucumber, diced
- 1/4 cup chopped fresh cilantro
- 2 tablespoons lime juice
- 1 tablespoon olive oil
- 1 tablespoon honey
- 1 teaspoon minced garlic
- Optional: red pepper flakes, for heat

Instructions:

1. Preheat your grill to medium-high heat.
2. Season the steaks generously with salt and pepper.
3. In a small bowl, combine diced cucumber, chopped cilantro, lime juice, olive oil, honey, minced garlic, and red pepper flakes if using. Mix well to combine.
4. Grill the steaks to your desired level of doneness, about 4-5 minutes per side for medium-rare, depending on thickness.
5. Remove the steaks from the grill and let them rest for a few minutes before serving.
6. Serve the grilled steaks topped with cucumber-cilantro salsa.
7. Enjoy this flavorful and refreshing dish!

Nutritional Values (Approximate, per serving):

- Calories: 300-350 kcal
- Protein: 25-30 grams
- Fat: 15-20 grams

- Carbohydrates: 5-8 grams

- Dietary Fiber: 1-2 grams

- Sugars: 3-5 grams

Classic Pot Roast:

Prep	**Time:**	15	minutes
Cook	**Time:**	3-4	hours

Servings: 6

Ingredients:

- 1 (3-4 lb) beef chuck roast

- Salt and pepper, to taste

- 2 tablespoons vegetable oil

- 1 onion, sliced

- 4 carrots, peeled and cut into chunks

- 4 potatoes, peeled and cut into chunks

- 2 cloves garlic, minced

- 2 cups beef broth

- 1 cup red wine (optional)

- 2 sprigs fresh thyme

- 2 sprigs fresh rosemary

Instructions:

1. Preheat your oven to 325°F (165°C).

2. Season the beef chuck roast generously with salt and pepper.

3. Heat vegetable oil in a large Dutch oven over medium-high heat. Sear the beef roast on all sides until browned, about 3-4 minutes per side. Remove the roast from the pot and set aside.

4. In the same pot, add sliced onion, carrot chunks, potato chunks, and minced garlic. Cook for 3-4 minutes until vegetables start to soften.

5. Return the beef roast to the pot. Pour in beef broth and red wine (if using). Add fresh thyme and rosemary sprigs.

6. Cover the pot with a lid and transfer it to the preheated oven.

7. Roast for 3-4 hours, or until the beef is fork-tender and the vegetables are cooked through.

8. Remove the pot roast from the oven and let it rest for a few minutes before slicing.

9. Serve slices of pot roast with the cooked vegetables and pan juices.

10. Enjoy this comforting and hearty classic pot roast!

Nutritional Values (Approximate, per serving):

- Calories: 400-500 kcal

- Protein: 30-40 grams

- Fat: 20-30 grams

- Carbohydrates: 15-20 grams

- Dietary Fiber: 3-5 grams

- Sugars: 3-5 grams

30 DAYS MEAL PLAN

Week 1:

Day 1:

- Breakfast: Veggie and Hummus Wrap
- Lunch: Lentil Soup with Whole Grain Bread Rolls
- Dinner: Vegetable Curry with Brown Rice

Day 2:

- Breakfast: Cucumber-Dill Cabbage Salad with Lemon Dressing
- Lunch: French Onion Soup
- Dinner: Roasted Chicken Thighs with Sweet Potatoes and Green Beans

Day 3:

- Breakfast: Blueberry-Pineapple Smoothie
- Lunch: Chicken and Vegetable Skewers with Brown Rice Pilaf
- Dinner: Eggplant Parmesan with Mixed Green Salad

Day 4:

- Breakfast: Leaf Lettuce and Carrot Salad with Balsamic Vinaigrette
- Lunch: Fish and Seafood Entrées
- Dinner: Ratatouille served over Quinoa

Day 5:

- Breakfast: Strawberry-Watercress Salad with Almond Dressing
- Lunch: Cream of Watercress Soup
- Dinner: Grilled Steak with Cucumber-Cilantro Salsa

Day 6:

- Breakfast: Farfalle Confetti Salad
- Lunch: Tuna and White Bean Salad
- Dinner: Shrimp Scampi Linguine

Day 7:

- Breakfast: Sweet and Spicy Kettle Corn
- Lunch: Baked Cod with Cucumber-Dill Salsa
- Dinner: Herb-Crusted Baked Haddock

Week 2:

Day 8:

- Breakfast: Veggie and Hummus Wrap
- Lunch: Lentil Soup with Whole Grain Bread Rolls
- Dinner: Vegetable Curry with Brown Rice

Day 9:

- Breakfast: Cucumber-Dill Cabbage Salad with Lemon Dressing
- Lunch: French Onion Soup
- Dinner: Roasted Chicken Thighs with Sweet Potatoes and Green Beans

Day 10:

- Breakfast: Blueberry-Pineapple Smoothie
- Lunch: Chicken and Vegetable Skewers with Brown Rice Pilaf
- Dinner: Eggplant Parmesan with Mixed Green Salad

Day 11:

- Breakfast: Leaf Lettuce and Carrot Salad with Balsamic Vinaigrette
- Lunch: Fish and Seafood Entrées
- Dinner: Ratatouille served over Quinoa

Day 12:

- Breakfast: Strawberry-Watercress Salad with Almond Dressing
- Lunch: Cream of Watercress Soup
- Dinner: Grilled Steak with Cucumber-Cilantro Salsa

Day 13:

- Breakfast: Farfalle Confetti Salad
- Lunch: Tuna and White Bean Salad

- Dinner: Shrimp Scampi Linguine

Day 14:

- Breakfast: Sweet and Spicy Kettle Corn
- Lunch: Baked Cod with Cucumber-Dill Salsa
- Dinner: Herb-Crusted Baked Haddock

Week 3:

Day 15:

- Breakfast: Leaf Lettuce and Asparagus Salad with Raspberries
- Lunch: Turkey-Bulgur Soup
- Dinner: Herb Pesto Tuna

Day 16:

- Breakfast: Waldorf Salad
- Lunch: Ground Beef and Rice Soup
- Dinner: Persian Chicken

Day 17:

- Breakfast: Couscous Salad with Spicy Citrus Dressing
- Lunch: Shrimp Scampi Linguine
- Dinner: Pesto Pork Chops

Day 18:

- Breakfast: Tabbouleh
- Lunch: Beef Stir-Fry with Broccoli and Bell Peppers
- Dinner: Pork Souvlaki

Day 19:

- Breakfast: Ginger Beef Salad
- Lunch: Lentil Soup with Whole Grain Bread Rolls
- Dinner: Roasted Beef Stew

Day 20:

- Breakfast: Chicken Stir-Fry

- Lunch: French Onion Soup
- Dinner: Baked Cod with Herbed Cauliflower Rice

Day 21:

- Breakfast: Mediterranean Chickpea Salad
- Lunch: Chicken and Vegetable Kebabs with Brown Rice Pilaf
- Dinner: Chicken Curry

Week 4:

Day 22:

- Breakfast: Veggie and Hummus Wrap
- Lunch: Herb-Crusted Baked Haddock
- Dinner: Cucumber-Wrapped Vegetable Rolls

Day 23:

- Breakfast: Leaf Lettuce and Carrot Salad with Balsamic Vinaigrette
- Lunch: Tuna and White Bean Salad
- Dinner: Sweet Glazed Salmon

Day 24:

- Breakfast: French Onion Soup
- Lunch: Roasted Chicken Thighs with Sweet Potatoes and Green Beans
- Dinner: Pesto Pork Chops

Day 25:

- Breakfast: Tabbouleh
- Lunch: Chicken Stir-Fry
- Dinner: Grilled Calamari with Lemon and Herbs

Day 26:

- Breakfast: Waldorf Salad
- Lunch: Vegetable Curry with Brown Rice
- Dinner: Sweet and Sour Meat Loaf

Day 27:

- Breakfast: Strawberry-Watercress Salad with Almond Dressing
- Lunch: Lentil Soup with Whole Grain Bread Rolls
- Dinner: Classic Pot Roast

Day 28:

- Breakfast: Couscous Salad with Spicy Citrus Dressing
- Lunch: Baked Cod with Cucumber-Dill Salsa
- Dinner: Open-Faced Beef Stir-Up

GLOSSARY

1. **Blanching**: A cooking process where food, usually vegetables or fruits, is briefly immersed in boiling water, then removed and placed in ice water to halt the cooking process. It helps retain color and texture.

2. **Braise**: A cooking method where food, often meat, is first browned in fat, then cooked slowly in a covered pot with a small amount of liquid (such as broth or wine) until tender.

3. **Broil**: To cook food directly under high heat, usually in an oven or grill. It helps to brown the surface of the food quickly.

4. **Deglaze**: To add liquid, such as broth or wine, to a pan in which meat has been cooked to dissolve and loosen the browned bits of food stuck to the bottom. It adds flavor to sauces and gravies.

5. **Dredge**: To coat food, such as meat or fish, with flour, breadcrumbs, or cornmeal before cooking. It helps to create a crispy outer layer when cooked.

6. **Julienne**: A knife-cutting technique where food, typically vegetables, is cut into thin, uniform matchstick shapes.

7. **Marinate**: To soak food, usually meat or vegetables, in a seasoned liquid mixture (marinade) to add flavor and tenderize before cooking.

8. **Poach**: To cook food gently in barely simmering liquid, such as water or broth. It's often used for delicate foods like eggs or fish.

9. **Sauté**: To cook food quickly in a small amount of fat over high heat, using a shallow pan. It's a common method for cooking vegetables or meat.

10. **Simmer**: To cook food gently in liquid at a temperature just below boiling. It's often used for soups, stews, and sauces.

11. **Sear**: To brown the surface of food quickly over high heat, usually meat, before finishing cooking by another method. It helps to develop flavor and texture.

12. **Zest**: The colored outer part of citrus fruit peel, used as a flavoring in cooking. It's obtained by scraping or cutting away the outer layer of the peel without including the bitter white pith.